T0201157

Perform Operative Procedures in Obstetrics and Gynaecology

how to
Perform Operative Procedures in Obstetrics and Gynaecology

Edited by

Wai Yoong, MBBCh, MD, FRCOG
Consultant Obstetrician and Urogynaecologist
North Middlesex University Hospital London;
Honorary Senior Lecturer, University College London, London, UK;
Associate Professor
St George's International School of Medicine, Grenada, West Indies

Abha Govind, MBBS, FFSRH, FRCOG
Consultant Obstetrician and Gynaecologist
North Middlesex University Hospital London;
Honorary Senior Lecturer, University College London, London, UK;
Associate Professor
St George's International School of Medicine, Grenada, West Indies

Wasim Lodhi, MBBS, PGCert MedEd, FRCOG
Consultant Obstetrician and Gynaecologist
North Middlesex University Hospital London;
Honorary Senior Lecturer, University College London, London, UK;
Associate Professor
St George's International School of Medicine, Grenada, West Indies

WILEY Blackwell

This edition first published 2020
© 2020 John Wiley & Sons Ltd

All rights reserved. No part of this publication may be reproduced, stored in a retrieval system, or transmitted, in any form or by any means, electronic, mechanical, photocopying, recording or otherwise, except as permitted by law. Advice on how to obtain permission to reuse material from this title is available at http://www.wiley.com/go/permissions.

The right of Wai Yoong, Abha Govind, and Wasim Lodhi to be identified as the authors of the editorial material in this work has been asserted in accordance with law.

Registered Office(s)
John Wiley & Sons, Inc., 111 River Street, Hoboken, NJ 07030, USA
John Wiley & Sons Ltd, The Atrium, Southern Gate, Chichester, West Sussex, PO19 8SQ, UK

Editorial Office
9600 Garsington Road, Oxford, OX4 2DQ, UK

For details of our global editorial offices, customer services, and more information about Wiley products visit us at www.wiley.com.

Wiley also publishes its books in a variety of electronic formats and by print-on-demand. Some content that appears in standard print versions of this book may not be available in other formats.

Limit of Liability/Disclaimer of Warranty
The contents of this work are intended to further general scientific research, understanding, and discussion only and are not intended and should not be relied upon as recommending or promoting scientific method, diagnosis, or treatment by physicians for any particular patient. In view of ongoing research, equipment modifications, changes in governmental regulations, and the constant flow of information relating to the use of medicines, equipment, and devices, the reader is urged to review and evaluate the information provided in the package insert or instructions for each medicine, equipment, or device for, among other things, any changes in the instructions or indication of usage and for added warnings and precautions. While the publisher and authors have used their best efforts in preparing this work, they make no representations or warranties with respect to the accuracy or completeness of the contents of this work and specifically disclaim all warranties, including without limitation any implied warranties of merchantability or fitness for a particular purpose. No warranty may be created or extended by sales representatives, written sales materials or promotional statements for this work. The fact that an organization, website, or product is referred to in this work as a citation and/or potential source of further information does not mean that the publisher and authors endorse the information or services the organization, website, or product may provide or recommendations it may make. This work is sold with the understanding that the publisher is not engaged in rendering professional services. The advice and strategies contained herein may not be suitable for your situation. You should consult with a specialist where appropriate. Further, readers should be aware that websites listed in this work may have changed or disappeared between when this work was written and when it is read. Neither the publisher nor authors shall be liable for any loss of profit or any other commercial damages, including but not limited to special, incidental, consequential, or other damages.

Library of Congress Cataloging-in-Publication Data
Names: Yoong, Wai, editor. | Govind, Abha, editor. | Lodhi, Wasim, editor.
Title: How to perform operative procedures in obstetrics and gynaecology / edited by Wai Yoong, Abha Govind, Wasim Lodhi.
Description: Hoboken, NJ : John Wiley & Sons, 2020. | Includes bibliographical references and index.
Identifiers: LCCN 2020001833 (print) | LCCN 2020001834 (ebook) | ISBN 9781118672884 (paperback) | ISBN 9781119690887 (adobe pdf) | ISBN 9781119690870 (epub)
Subjects: MESH: Gynecologic Surgical Procedures–methods | Obstetric Surgical Procedures–methods
Classification: LCC RG101 (print) | LCC RG101 (ebook) | NLM WP 660 | DDC 618.1–dc23
LC record available at https://lccn.loc.gov/2020001833
LC ebook record available at https://lccn.loc.gov/2020001834

Cover Design: Wiley
Cover Image: Courtesy of Wai Yoong and Abha Govind

Set in 8.5/12pt HelveticaNeueLight by SPi Global, Pondicherry, India
Printed and bound in Singapore by Markono Print Media Pte Ltd

10 9 8 7 6 5 4 3 2 1

Contents

Contributors

Katie Andersen, MRCOG
ST7 Obstetrics and Gynaecology trainee
Whittington Hospital, London, UK

Rosalind Aughwane, PhD, MRCOG
ST5 Obstetrics and Gynaecology trainee
Homerton University Hospital, London, UK

Charlotte Austen, MRCOG
ST5 Obstetrics and Gynaecology trainee
Barnet Hospital, Barnet, UK

Natasha Barbaneagra, MRCOG
Consultant Obstetrician and Gynaecologist
Barnet Hospital, Barnet, UK

Joan Baqer, MRCOG
Post CESR Trust Obstetrician and
Gynaecologist
North Middlesex University Hospital
London, UK

Sayantana Das, MRCOG
ST6 Obstetrics and Gynaecology trainee
The Royal London Hospital – Barts Health
NHS Trust, London, UK

Roberto De Martino
British Airways Training Captain
British Airways Flight Training, BA Global
Learning Academy, Technical Block A
Vanguard Way, London Heathrow Airport
Longford, UK

Dhanuson Dharmasena, MRCOG
ST6 Obstetrics and Gynaecology trainee
North Middlesex University Hospital
London, UK

Jane Ding, PhD, MRCOG
ST6 Obstetrics and Gynaecology trainee
Barking, Havering and Redbridge
University Hospitals, Romford, UK

Rajvinder Khasriya, PhD, MRCOG
Consultant Urogynaecologist
Whittington Hospital, London, UK

Ciara MacKenzie, MRCOG
ST5 Obstetrics and Gynaecology trainee
University College Hospital – Elizabeth
Garrett Anderson, London, UK

Maud Nauta, MBBCh, MRCGP
General Practitioner
Camden Health Improvement Practice
The Margarete Centre, London, UK

Christina Neophytou, MBBCh
ST1 Obstetrics and Gynaecology trainee
North Middlesex University Hospital
London, UK

Mark Ponnusamy
British Airways Senior First Flight Officer
British Airways Flight Training, BA Global
Learning Academy, Technical Block A
Vanguard Way, London Heathrow Airport
Longford, UK

Sophie Relph, MRCOG
Senior Registrar, North East London
Deanery and Clinical Research Fellow
Department of Women's and Children's
Health, King's College London
The Strand, London, UK

Beena Subba, FRCOG
Consultant Obstetrician and Gynaecologist
North Middlesex University Hospital
London, UK

Foreword

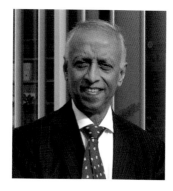

This practical procedures-oriented text book and videos in the companion website is a must read/see book for every trainee and junior consultant in obstetrics and gynaecology. The book has 23 chapters with excellent illustrative photographs and figures of the procedures. The companion website has 19 accompanied videos with a commentary that covers the spectrum of common procedures in obstetrics and gynaecology. The videos are brief to the point and of high quality. The accompanying commentary explains every step of the procedure.

The text book is divided into three parts: Part I, Basic concepts with six chapters; Part II, Obstetrics with four chapters, and Part III, Gynaecology with 13 chapters. Part I covers six important basic aspects of any surgical discipline, i.e. consent, WHO safety surgical check list, understanding human factors in obstetrics and gynaecology, surgical instruments, surgical positioning, and sutures and needles. These are

"must read" chapters for any O&G specialist. The videos on surgical instruments, surgical positioning, and sutures and needles explain the basic aspects of surgery for easy visual understanding.

Part II covers two important common operative procedures in obstetrics: Assisted vaginal delivery and Caesarean section followed by two rare but essential procedures of uterine compression sutures for uterine atony and cervical cerclage, both elective and emergency.

Part III covers 12 commonly performed gynaecological operative procedures. The chapters and accompanying videos cover simple procedures such as manual vacuum aspiration and surgical management of miscarriage, female sterilisation by laparoscopic and hysteroscopic approaches to more complex procedures including abdominal and vaginal hysterectomy.

The authors of the chapters have explained the operations in simple language in a stepwise manner with illustrative photographs and figures so that the contents are easily understood by the reader. The text covers more important useful points than can be shared in the video. The chapters also provide a list of further reading materials that have been carefully selected. Complementing the written illustrated chapters with visual portrayal by videos is a brilliant way of enabling the juniors to become familiar with these procedures. The editors are well known and accomplished trainers of practical procedures in obstetrics and gynaecology for several years. They have distilled their thoughts in editing the chapters and videos. The editors and authors should be congratulated for their effort in producing this valuable text book and companion website of complimentary videos.

March 2020

Sir Sabaratnam Arulkumaran
Professor Emeritus of Obstetrics &
Gynaecology
Past President – RCOG,
FIGO & BMA

Editors' Biographies

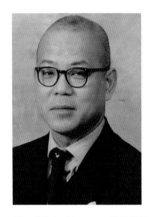

Mr Wai Yoong (MBBCh Belf, MD London, FRCOG UK) is a consultant Obstetrician and Urogynaecologist at North Middlesex University Hospital London and an Honorary Senior Lecturer at University College London and Associate Professor at St George's International School of Medicine. He received his general O&G training in Birmingham and London and completed a Urogynaecology Fellowship in Sydney, Australia. He is the senior organiser of the RCOG Masterclass in Management of Massive Obstetric Haemorrhage and senior founder trustee of Haemorrhage After Childbirth Foundation, a charity dedicated to teaching skills to doctors and midwives on how to manage obstetric haemorrhage. He was the past RCOG National Convenor of Basic Practical Skills Course and is on the Editorial Board of The Obstetrician and Gynaecologist (TOG), as well as the Journal of Obstetrics and Gynaecology. He leads a team of clinicians partnering with British Airways Flight Training to deliver a collaborative aviation-healthcare Human Factors training course using flight simulators and interactive facilitation to reduce medical errors (see: https://www.britishairways.com/en-gb/baft/human-factors/ClinicalHumanFactors).

In 2014, he was awarded the Sims Black Travelling Professorship by the Royal College of Obstetricians and Gynaecologists to teach Basic Surgical Skills and PPH management in Jordan. In 2018, he was given the Bernhard Baron Travelling Scholarship to learn about the surgical management of morbidly adherent placenta with Professor Jose Palacios in Buenas Aires, Argentina. He has published 129 papers in peer review journals on subjects such as vaginal surgery, surgical management of PPH, human factors, neuromodulation and enhanced recovery.

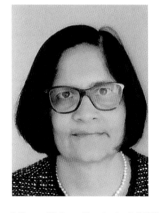

Miss Abha Govind (MBBS, FFSRH, FRCOG) is a consultant Obstetrician and Gynaecologist at North Middlesex University Hospital London and an Honorary Senior Lecturer at University College London and Associate Professor at St George's International School of Medicine. Her specialist interests include high risk obstetrics, obstetric ultrasound scanning, reproductive endocrinology and sexual & reproductive health.

She has held educational and management posts including deanery College tutor, MBBS, DRCOG and MRCOG part 2 examiner, faculty trainer for DFSRH, deanery ATSM preceptor in fetal medicine and abortion care, lead clinician & lead for clinical governance & risk management in maternity. She has been faculty on the RCOG EMQ and SBA writing, MRCOG Part 2 written and MRCOG Final preparation OSCE at the RCOG. She has also taught on the RCOG Virtual Revision Course since its inception in 2012 and Basic Practical Skills course.

She has offered a weekly family planning service for the Haringey PCT since 2000 and has helped train several GPs & hospital doctors, enabling them to attain a diploma in sexual and reproductive health. In 2014 she was the winner of the North Middlesex Hospital Staff award for best team providing exemplary care for HIV in pregnancy. In 2017 she was nominated and was runner up for North Middlesex individual Staff Awards in the category of outstanding contribution to patient care. She has 41 publications in peer reviewed journals and has contributed to book chapters on topics relevant to feto-maternal medicine, contraception and sexual health.

Gynaecologist from North Middlesex University Hospital with a special interest in outpatient operative hysteroscopy, which he developed as a Visiting Clinical Fellow at the University of Naples Federico II, Italy. He is a co-organiser of the RCOG Masterclass in Massive Obstetric Haemorrhage workshops and has facilitated at Harassment and Undermining workshops nationally. He is heavily involved with the Royal College of Obstetricians and Gynaecologists and is the past National Convenor of Basic Practical Skills (BPS) course as well as Chairperson of the RCOG Pakistan Liaison Group. He is faculty member of the MRCOG parts I, II and III courses as well as being an examiner of the MRCOG part III course. He is a founder trustee of Haemorrhage After Childbirth Foundation, a charity dedicated to teaching skills to doctors and midwives on how to manage obstetric haemorrhage. He is a certified Human Factors Instructor and faculty member of the British Airways Flight Training Human Factors team which teaches Crew Resource Management to clinicians and healthcare professionals.

Disclaimer

This book represents an effort to help and understand commonly performed procedures in obstetrics and gynaecology. The editors acknowledge that the techniques shown here are not the only way of performing the operations.

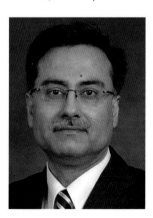

Mr Wasim Lodhi (MBBS FRCOG PGCert MedEd) is a consultant Obstetrician and

Acknowledgements

The exact date that we were first commissioned to produce this innovative video book is shrouded in the mists of time, but I am pleased that following a long gestation we have finally arrived at the end of our journey. NHS workload and distractions of other projects stalled our progress but, thankfully, the addition of Abha Govind as co-editor lent fresh impetus and urgency to complete this work. I am grateful to Wasim Lodhi for his friendship and support throughout the project. Ivano and Walter from Ionised Media have been very patient in redrafting the various versions of the video footages.

This video book is to serve as an aide-de-memoire for commonly seen surgical procedures at MRCOG and senior registrar level and we hope that this will serve as a useful audio-visual tool for training. I would like to thank the contributors, most of whom had worked at one time or another in our unit at North Middlesex University Hospital NHS Trust. Lastly, I would like to acknowledge the unstinting support and encouragement of my wife, Maud, and teenagers, Helienke, Douwejan and Janna, in seeing this video book to final fruition.

Wai Yoong

I would like to thank all the women who willingly consented to making this book happen. My sincere thanks to my colleagues Wai and Wasim who made this project possible and let me be a part of the journey. I would also like to thank my parents, Kamla and Har Govind for their inspiration and my husband Devesh for his unwavering support and belief in me.

Abha Govind

It was a long journey from the conception to the actual delivery of this book. Having embarked on this journey of production of a video book to help our junior colleagues preparing for MRCOG examination, we had to alter our project to keep it updated and in line with the changes in the examination system trends of modern communication, i.e. electronic to fit in to the life of a busy trainee preparing for MRCOG examination.

I am grateful to my colleagues for their endless support and hard work in writing up various chapters. I am grateful to patients who graciously consented to let us record the procedures for teaching and training purposes. I am especially thankful to my colleague Wai Yoong for his enthusiasm and accepting the challenge to produce a first video book to help trainees prepare for the MRCOG examination and further. I can never thank enough our colleague Abha Govind for being extremely meticulous and organised in bringing everything together and giving a shape to this book. We are grateful to Wiley for their patience despite delays in our delivery of this book.

Lastly, I would like to thank my wife Zainab for her support by keeping my sons Zain and Mueez entertained while I was working on this project and was unable to give them time. This video book will be a lasting memory for them too.

Wasim Lodhi

About the Companion Website

This book is accompanied by a website:

www.wiley.com/go/yoong/obgyn

The website includes 20 detailed videos, with a voiceover, on how to perform specific obstetric and gynaecological procedures:

Chapter 4: Surgical instruments
Chapter 5: Surgical positioning
Chapter 6: Sutures
Chapter 7: Assisted vaginal delivery
Chapter 8: Caesarean section
Chapter 9: Uterine compression sutures for uterine atony
Chapter 10: Cervical cerclage
Chapter 11: Total abdominal hysterectomy
Chapter 12: Open myomectomy
Chapter 13: Hysteroscopic resection of fibroid
Chapter 14: Diagnostic laparoscopy

Chapter 15: Operative laparoscopy
Chapter 16: Laparoscopic salpingectomy for ectopic pregnancy
Chapter 17: Surgery for vaginal prolapse
Chapter 18: Vaginal hysterectomy
Chapter 19: Manchester repair
Chapter 20: Cone biopsy
Chapter 21: Rigid cystoscopy
Chapter 22: Evacuation of retained products of conception and manual vacuum aspiration
Chapter 23: Female sterilisation: the laparoscopic and hysteroscopic approaches

Note: There are no videos in Chapters 1–3.

PART I

Basic

1 Consent

Abha Govind

Overview

Obtaining consent and understanding its implications form an important part of a clinician's practice. This chapter discusses aspects of consent typically encountered by a clinician, including the recent Montgomery Ruling.

Introduction

In recent years, great emphasis has been placed on obtaining **consent** for surgical procedures to avoid litigation. This has become an integral part of clinical risk management and governance. Generally, consent should be obtained before any procedure. It is important to understand that a **competent adult** has the fundamental right to give, or withhold, consent to examination, investigation or treatment, founded on the moral principle of respect for autonomy. An **autonomous** person may decide what may or may not be done to her.

In **English civil law** deliberately touching another person without consent is called **battery,** which is punishable by law. Equally, patients can take out a **civil action** for **negligence** for not receiving enough information about a procedure, particularly if they have not been told enough about the **risks.** This could result in an action for damages, or even **criminal proceedings,** and potentially in a finding of a **serious professional misconduct** by a professional registration body, e.g. the General Medical Council (GMC).

Types of Consent

There are three different types of consent in everyday working practice. **Tacit** consent is when you tell a patient you want to take a blood test and she holds out her arm whilst you put a needle in and take the blood sample. **Verbal** consent is when you ask a patient if you can do a vaginal examination and she says yes and allows the procedure. Finally, **written** consent should be taken for all **invasive procedures**, those involving **risk** and where regional or **general anaesthesia** is required. It is not absolutely necessary to defend an action for assault/battery but it affords **documentary evidence.** If an action is brought several years after the event, the judge may prefer the patient's evidence over that of the practitioner, if

How to Perform Operative Procedures in Obstetrics and Gynaecology, First Edition.
Edited by Wai Yoong, Abha Govind, and Wasim Lodhi.
© 2020 John Wiley & Sons Ltd. Published 2020 by John Wiley & Sons Ltd.
Companion website: www.wiley.com/go/yoong/obgyn

a signed and witnessed consent form cannot be produced.

What Makes Consent Valid?

Consent must be given **voluntarily,** without coercion, by a woman who is **fully informed** about the procedure or investigation in question, and who has capacity. It is not valid if she agrees to an operation without full knowledge. If possible, **visual or written aids** can be used to help, and an **interpreter** should be used if needed. Consideration also needs to be given to patients with learning difficulties.

When Should You Obtain Consent?

Ideally, well in advance so that the patient has time to ask questions. It is good practice to obtain consent in **outpatient** clinics, then **confirm** consent prior to the procedure. In certain cases, women are listed for theatre within days of being seen in clinic (e.g. women with cancer) and in this instance it is important that the woman has been given the opportunity to reflect on the procedure and to ask questions. The GMC recommends an appropriate **cooling off** period before signing.

How Long Is Consent Valid for?

If a woman consents to a procedure, generally it is assumed that this consent is valid **indefinitely.** However, in a few situations consent may need to be **reconfirmed,** e.g. if the patient's condition changes, if there is a long time period between signing and the procedure, or if the procedure has changed or new risks or side effects are known (DOH 2009).

Who Can Obtain Consent?

The responsibility for obtaining consent lies with the **clinician performing the operation.** Consent may not be valid if obtained by someone with inadequate knowledge of the procedure. If you are a junior trainee in this situation you have a duty to ensure you have the correct knowledge, and if you do not, refer the woman to another practitioner who does.

Fully Informed Consent

Ensure that your patient understands the **nature** of the condition, **intervention** and likely **benefits** and **risks** of the procedure for which the consent is proposed. She should also be told of the risks of the **procedure not being carried out.** When using consent forms in the UK, there is a space on the form to document any **procedures** that your patient **would not wish to have done.** For example, a person who is a **Jehovah's Witness** will not accept blood products, or a woman who wishes to retain her cervix with consent only for a subtotal hysterectomy.

Material Risk

These are defined as those to which a **reasonable person** in the patient's position would be likely to attach **significance.** It is an aspect of consent which has been contentious in terms of how much information regarding risks is given to patients. Several court cases have led to the current view that **as much information** as possible should be given to the patient.

The **'Bolam test'** is a defence to the charge of **negligence,** when a group of doctors within the same specialty agree that at the time they would have taken the same actions or decisions to the same standard (**Bolam v Friern Hospital Management Committee** (1957)). In the Sidaway case (**Sidaway v Board of Governors of the Bethlem Royal Hospital** (1985)), the patient was suffering from symptoms of nerve compression and underwent cord decompression. As a complication she suffered paraplegia, a recognised but uncommon complication (1–2%). This was not included in the consent. The patient reported negligence because of this but the court rejected the argument based on the Bolam test as other practitioners agreed it was not necessary to inform the patient of every risk. However, the House of Lords later concluded that a doctor has a duty to provide to their patients **sufficient information** for them to reach a **balanced judgement.** Since the **Sidaway** case, law courts are more willing to be critical of medical opinion, i.e. a clinician may be held accountable for an action being negligent or harmful, even if a body of professionals felt their action was reasonable according to the Bolam test.

Since the **Chester v Afshar** case (2004), it is now advised that when obtaining consent, practitioners should **inform** patients about **all significant** possible adverse outcomes. In this case, the patient sought advice from a neurosurgeon about their back pain and was advised to have an operation. This operation carried a 1–2% risk of **worsening the symptoms,** which the patient subsequently suffered but this was not discussed within the consent. Crucially, the court judged that the surgeon breached their duty as although the complication was not because of the surgeon's negligence during the operation, the link between omitting the risk during consent and the complication was causal – the claimant reported if they had been told of this risk they would have sought alternative advice or treatment (Chester v Afshar 2004). It is therefore imperative that practitioners should inform patients about **all significant possible adverse outcomes** and document this, and advise the patient if any intervention may result in a serious adverse outcome, even if the likelihood is very small (GMC 2008).

The law on consent has progressed from being **doctor led** to **patient focused.** When seeking consent to treatment, the question of whether the information given to a patient is adequate is judged from the perspective of a reasonable person in the patient's position. For the purposes of consent, the ruling from **Montgomery** replaces the previous tests founded in Bolam and refined in Sidaway. Doctors have a duty to take reasonable care to ensure that patients are aware of **'material risks'.**

Montgomery v Lanarkshire Health Board

Mrs Montgomery was a primigravida with type I diabetes who booked under consultant-led care in 1999. She was noted to have a large baby at her 36-week scan and was induced at 38 + 5 weeks of gestation. Although she expressed concerns about the size of the baby, the risk of shoulder dystocia (9–10% in diabetic mothers) was never discussed with her. Her consultant, who advised a vaginal delivery, defended her practice saying that in her estimation, 'the risk of a grave problem for the baby arising as a result of shoulder dystocia was very small (0.1%)'. The baby was delivered by forceps, but this was complicated by shoulder dystocia and there was a delay of 12 minutes between the delivery of the fetal head and body. Her son developed severe dyskinetic cerebral palsy as a result of hypoxia during delivery (Cheung et al. 2016). Her obstetrician had not disclosed the increased risk of this complication in vaginal delivery, despite Montgomery asking if the baby's size was a potential problem. Montgomery sued for negligence, arguing that, if she had known of the increased risk, she would have requested a Caesarean section. The Supreme Court of the UK announced judgement in her favour in

March 2015. The ruling overturned a previous decision by the House of Lords (Sidaway v Board of Governors of the Bethlem Royal Hospital 1985; Heywood 2015). It established that, rather than being a matter for clinical judgment to be assessed by professional medical opinion, a patient should be told whatever they want to know, not what the doctor thinks they should be told.

The judgement therefore means that doctors must share all such material risks, as well as any to which it would be reasonable for them to think the individual patient would attach significance. Although Montgomery changed the legal position, the principle of involving patients in their treatment and sharing information with them about risks has been in place for some time. The Medical Defence Union (**MDU)** has consistently been advising members to that effect for many years, and the **GMC** does the same in its guidance, entitled, '**Consent: doctors and patients making decisions togethe**r' (GMC 2008).

The practitioner should also bear in mind that their own perception of risk may differ to the woman's perception of risk, and so using terms which are clear and understandable is very important. For example, describing the likelihood of a complication as the likelihood of it affecting one person in a village, small town or large town.

Do Not Exceed the Authority Given by the Patient

Consent is given on the basis that the patient understands that any procedure in addition to the investigation or treatment described '… will only be carried out if it is necessary and in my best interest and can be justified for medical reasons' (DOH, consent Form 1). This covers what becomes necessary during the operation for the preservation of the patient's life or health. It **does not** allow the surgeon to **contravene** the **expressed wish** of the patient and to undertake albeit well-meaning procedures for which the patient has not given consent. She is entitled to be told what procedures may reasonably be expected to be carried out. It would be wise to tell the patient whilst consenting her for general anaesthesia, if an analgesics suppository is to be inserted. In 1995, the GMC made a finding of serious professional misconduct against an anaesthetist who inserted the suppository without giving such a warning. In 1997, a gynaecologist was accused of **serious professional misconduct** by the GMC after he removed the ovaries of a patient during a routine operation for a hysterectomy. He believed the findings at the operation justified removal of the ovaries, but he had not obtained specific consent for their removal (Dyer 2000).

With **medical students,** it is important that consent is taken for procedure or examinations which are performed by students or trainees solely for their own education or training.

Establishing Capacity

The Mental Capacity Act (MCA) **assumes** that all adults have **capacity** until proven otherwise (Mental Capacity Act 2005). In order to be sure your patient has capacity to consent there are four important principles: she must **understand** the information, **retain** information long enough to decide, be able to **weigh up** the available information and be able to **communicate her decision** back. A person lacks capacity if they have a disturbance of mind or brain which means they cannot make a specific decision. It is important to remember that capacity is decision- and time-specific. A woman may not have capacity to decide whether to have a hysterectomy for menorrhagia, but can consent to have a blood test to test her haemoglobin. It is important that capacity is not confused with a practitioner's impression that a decision is incorrect or against medical advice.

Mental Capacity Act

There are **five key principles** to the law relating to the MCA (2005). You must **presume** patient has **capacity** and if you doubt that they have capacity, then you should prove that they lack this. Every effort should be made to support the patient making their own decisions. This may mean simplifying or translating the information as appropriate. One must respect the patient's autonomy to make their own decision, even if you personally think the **decision is unwise.** Where a patient has no capacity, the concept of **best interests** comes into play. When a decision about what a women's best interests may be needs to be taken, a practitioner should seek another senior practitioner's **opinion** and may need **legal advice**. In some instances, an **Independent Mental Capacity Advocate** (IMCA**)** may have a role to play. Finally, whatever action you take it must be least restrictive of the patient's human rights.

When a Patient Lacks Capacity

In line with the MCA (2005), when a person lacks capacity, a health professional must **act in their best interests** and choose the **least restrictive options.** In acting in the patient's best interest, the health professional can take into account the person's **past and present wishes** and feelings, including relevant **written statement** made by her when she had capacity.

Apart from healthcare professionals, there are only two other parties who may make decisions on a patient's behalf. The first is someone with **lasting power of attorney** (MCA 2005), which is a person nominated by the patient, when she had capacity, who will make decisions on her behalf when she lacks capacity. Alternatively, the court can appoint an **IMCA,** whose role is to act in the best interest of patient. An IMCA can weigh up the information an make a decision in the best interest of patient.

Furthermore, when considering decisions which need to be made about a patient who lacks capacity, the practitioners must consult any **advanced directives** that may exist. A woman can make a decision in advance to refuse treatment, which is applicable for a time in the future when she does not have capacity. An advanced directive can be withdrawn by the patient at any time, as long as they retain capacity at the time of withdrawing it.

Right to Refuse Consent

A **competent adult** has the right to refuse treatment even if others, including doctors, believe that the refusal is neither in their best interests nor reasonable.

One case illustrating the right of a competent adult to refuse medical treatment is the case concerning a schizophrenic patient who suffered persecutory delusions and believed himself to be a doctor of international repute. This patient had refused to give consent for the amputation of his leg which had become gangrenous. The patient was considered by the judge to **have capacity** to make treatment decisions on his own behalf. This case also upholds the principle that mental illness does not automatically call a patient's capacity into question **(Re C. Adult: refusal of treatment 1994)**.

Consent Forms

The Department of Health has produced **four** different consent forms for use in practice in the UK. **Form 1** is consent by **competent adults or Gillick competent** child for general or local anaesthetic. This is the form generally used for consent, e.g. laparoscopy under general anaesthetic (GA). **Form 2** is consent by a **parent for a child** or young person less than 16 years of age. **Form 3** is used when **consciousness is not impaired** or no anaesthetic is needed, e.g. outpatient hysteroscopy or treatment in the colposcopy department. **Form 4** is used when an adult is unable to consent or in **adults without capacity**.

Special Situations

If a woman wishes to undergo a permanent form of contraception, e.g. **sterilisation,** it is important to discuss all risks and benefits with her. It is advisable to give the patient a cooling off period between consenting for the sterilisation and the procedure. It is important to stress that the **decision** for sterilisation **lies with the woman** and not with any partner she may have. When consenting for a **termination of pregnancy,** the decision lies solely with the woman; however, it is good practice to discuss with the patient's partner where relevant and to take into account their thoughts and views.

Fraser and Gillick Competence

Fraser guidelines and Gillick competence relate to issues of consent around children. Initially, these guidelines related to capacity and consent surrounding **contraception and child protection** issues. However, the Gillick case and subsequent Fraser guidelines are now used more widely to establish if a child under the age of 16 has the **maturity and capacity** to make a decision about their care and understand the implications of the decision.

Gillick competence is used to assess whether a child, 16 years or younger, is able to consent to his or her own medical treatment without the need for parental permission or knowledge.

The Gillick case involved a mother who took her local health authority to court to prevent them from giving contraceptive advice and treatment to girls under the age of 16 **(Gillick v West Norfolk and Wisbech AHA 1986)**. It was ruled that children who have sufficient understanding and intelligence to enable them to understand fully what is involved in a proposed intervention will also have the capacity to consent to that intervention. This is sometimes described as being **'Gillick competent'**.

Lord Fraser concluded that the doctor would be justified in proceeding without parental consent/or even knowledge if the girl, under 16 years of age, **understood** his advice.

Finally, recording video footages or images of the pelvis at operation (to form part of the operation record) is allowed but consent is needed if these are used for teaching purposes or publication.

Summary

- A **valid consent** shows it is allowed and that you are doing what is agreed.
- A legally recognised consent is one that is **fully informed** and given **without coercion.**
- Before taking consent, ascertain that the woman is **competent,** i.e. she can understand, retain, weigh the pros and cons and is able to communicate the information back.
- **Assume** all women over the age of 16 years have the **capacity** to give consent unless proven otherwise.

- A **Fraser competent** child is able to give voluntary and valid consent.
- Inform women of all **common and potentially serious risks** with due care and formality.
- The **Mental Capacity Act 2005** is used when patients lack capacity.
- Refer to **any advanced directives** when making decisions in those without capacity.
- In **emergencies** doctors must act in the **best interest** of the patient who is unable to consent.

Further Reading

Bolam v Friern Hospital Management Committee (1957). 1 WLR 5826. https://en.wikipedia.org/wiki/Bolam_v_Friern_Hospital_Management_Committee.

Chester v Afshar (2004). UKHL 41. https://publications.parliament.uk/pa/ld200304/ldjudgmt/jd041014/cheste-1.htm.

Cheung, E., Goodyear, G., and Yoong, W. (2016). TOG Medicolegal update on consent: 'The Montgomery Ruling'. https://obgyn.onlinelibrary.wiley.com/doi/epdf/10.1111/tog.12303.

DoH Guidance (2009). Reference guide to consent for examination or treatment (second edition) [https://www.gov.uk/government/publications/reference-guide-to-consent-for-examination-or-treatment-second-edition].

Dyer, C. (2000). Gynaecologist cleared in hysterectomy case. *BMJ* 320 (7234): 535.

Gillick v West Norfolk and Wisbech AHA (1986). https://swarb.co.uk/gillick-v-west-norfolk-and-wisbech-area-health-authority-and-department-of-health-and-social-security-hl-17-oct-1985.

GMC (2008). Consent: patients and doctors making decisions together. https://www.gmc-uk.org/ethical-guidance/ethical-guidance-for-doctors/consent.

Heywood, R. (2015). RIP Sidaway: patient-oriented disclosure—a standard worth waiting for? Montgomery v Lanarkshire Health Board UKSC 11. *Med Law Rev.* 23: 455–466. doi:https://doi.org/10.1093/medlaw/fwv024 pmid:26023076.

MDU Services Ltd (2018). Montgomery and informed consent. https://www.themdu.com/guidance-and-advice/guides/montgomery-and-informed-consent.

Medical Protection Society (2015). New judgement on patient consent. http://www.medicalprotection.org/uk/for-members/news/news/2015/03/20/new-judgment-on-patient-consent.

Mental Capacity Act (2005). Office of Public Guardian (2018). Lasting Power of Attorney. https://www.gov.uk/government/publications/make-a-lasting-power-of-attorney.

Montgomery v Lanarkshire Health Board (2015). UKSC 11. https://www.supremecourt.uk/cases/docs/uksc-2013-0136-judgment.pdf.

Re C (adult: refusal of medical treatment) (1994). 1 All ER 819 (QBD). www.cascaidr.org.uk/2017/03/22/re-c-adult-refusal-of-medical-treatment-1994-1-all-er-819-qbd.

Sidaway v Board of Governors of the Bethlem Royal Hospital (1985). AC 871. https://en.wikipedia.org/wiki/Sidaway_v_Board_of_Governors_of_the_Bethlem_Royal_Hospital.

2 WHO Surgical Safety Checklist

Sophie Relph and Wai Yoong

Overview

*There is no single remedy that will improve **surgical safety**. It requires reliable completion of a sequence of necessary steps not just by the surgeon, but by a team of healthcare professionals working together within a supportive health system for the benefit of the patient*

(World Alliance for Patient Safety 2008).

The World Health Organisation (WHO) Surgical Safety Checklist is a simple but thorough way of ensuring that surgical teams communicate relevant information effectively. Correct use of the checklist has already led to significant changes to morbidity and mortality rates in hospitals where the process is carried out. The authors explain the importance of introductions, briefings and the role of the WHO Surgical Safety Checklist in contemporary obstetrics and gynaecology theatre.

Introduction

An estimated 234 million operations are performed annually (Weiser et al. 2008), resulting in an estimated major **complication rate** of 3–17% and resultant **death rate** of 0.4–0.8%. Data suggests that at least half of all surgically-induced morbidity and mortality is avoidable (Gawande et al. 1999; Haynes et al. 2009) and surgical safety has become an international priority and a fundamental component of training in obstetrics and gynaecology.

In 2008, the WHO identified a simple set of surgical safety standards worldwide, which were applicable across all specialities. These were compiled into a **checklist** to be used in operating theatres across different countries. The initial pilot study was conducted in eight hospitals worldwide and demonstrated a fall in the surgically-associated death rate from 1.5 to 0.8% ($p = 0.003$), with a decrease in surgical complication rates from 11.0 to 7.0% ($p < 0.001$) after checklist implementation (Haynes et al. 2009).

In January 2009, the United Kingdom (UK) **National Patient Safety Agency** (NPSA) released a **Patient Safety Alert**. This

How to Perform Operative Procedures in Obstetrics and Gynaecology, First Edition.
Edited by Wai Yoong, Abha Govind, and Wasim Lodhi.
© 2020 John Wiley & Sons Ltd. Published 2020 by John Wiley & Sons Ltd.
Companion website: www.wiley.com/go/yoong/obgyn

required immediate action by Trusts nation-wide to introduce the checklist into their organisations for use in every surgical proce-dure (including those conducted under local anaesthesia) by October 2009 (NPSA, WHO 2009). In gynaecology, the WHO checklist (which can be modified by individual depart-ments) is used for all surgeries. In obstetrics, the WHO checklist has been adapted to also consider the safety of the baby or babies, as well as that of the mother.

Your Role

The surgical safety checklist is **everyone's responsibility** and requires the full atten-tion of the entire multi-disciplinary team allocated to the operating theatre. As a trainee, and frequently the primary surgeon for many operations, you must play an active role in the completion of the surgical safety checklist. Your safety as well as that of your team and your patient should remain your upmost concern at all times.

Starting the Day

Surgical safety checklists require the full attention and engagement of the **entire team**. Thus, the first task of the day is to get the team in the operating room without distractions and to conduct a short **brief-ing**. The aim of the briefing is to introduce each member of the team and outline a short plan for the day, including any changes to the list or prediction of any clini-cal or equipment problems. This also pro-vides an opportunity to **allocate a member** of the team with responsibility for conducting the WHO Surgical Safety Checklist for the duration of the list.

Why Are Team Introductions So Important?

Team introductions help team members to work together, **creating a shallow**

authority gradient so that a junior team member is empowered to point out to the senior consultant that the patient has chosen to conserve her ovaries, just as the latter may be about to perform bilateral oophorectomies during the abdominal hysterectomy.

Gynaecological Surgery – the 'Sign In'

The WHO Surgical Safety Checklist starts **before induction of anaesthesia** with the 'Sign In', which is usually completed in the anaesthetic room, and should be read out aloud (Figure 2.1). **Confirm the patient's identity** and check this against the wristband and consent form. Ask the patient **what procedure** they are expect-ing and verify the details and signature on the **consent form**. This avoids the likelihood of performing a laparoscopic sterilisation on a patient who only came in for a diagnos-tic laparoscopy and dye.

If applicable, check that the **surgical site** and **side** have been marked, using a non-soluble skin-marker which will not rub off with application of iodine/chlorhexidine. **'Wrong side surgery'** in a unilateral operation is a **'Never event'**! and this is especially important in endo-scopic surgery when video monitors may not be visualised by the rest of the surgi-cal team.

Ensure that the **anaesthetic equip-ment safety check** has been completed. If the patient has **known allergies,** check that the relevant allergy alert wristband in place. It is also vital for team members to be aware if the patient is allergic to latex, iodine or other routinely used adjunct surgi-cal bundle tools.

Is **additional monitoring equipment** or **other specific support** (such as a blood transfusion) required?

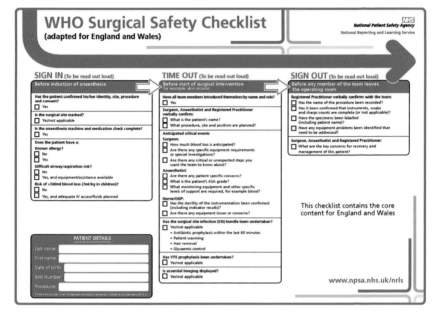

Figure 2.1 WHO surgical safety checklist.

Finally, for the anaesthetist, has the patient's American Society of Anesthesiology **(ASA) grade** been noted?

The 'Sign In' section of the form must then be authorised and dated by the responsible healthcare professional and induction of anaesthesia can begin.

Maternity Cases – The 'Sign In'

This form is only used for Caesarean section (CS) and the main difference with the Maternity 'Sign In' is that the woman is usually awake throughout the procedure, regional anaesthesia being commonly used, and that the safety of mother and fetus must be considered. The checklist should be **read aloud** after the arrival of the woman and the midwife into theatre. The same identity, allergy and anaesthetic confirmations are required and the **category of CS** is then documented on the form.

The following points are more specific to the CS checklist:

• Is a **difficult airway** anticipated, in case of intubation?
• Are **blood products** required and, if so, are those blood products available on the labour ward? Maternal death secondary to post-partum haemorrhage following Caesarean section is also considered a **'Never event'**.
• Has **appropriate antacid** prophylaxis been given?
• Is the **resuscitaire check** complete?
• Are the **neonatal team** needed?

The 'Time Out' usually follows immediately after in maternity cases, but is detailed in a later section.

Gynaecological Surgery – The 'Time Out'

This part of the checklist is completed when the patient is in theatre, before starting the skin incision. **All team members are** invited to introduce themselves by name and role. This introduction should be repeated every time a new member joins the team. **Confirm the patient's name** by comparing the wristband to the consent form. The lead surgeon will be asked **to verify procedure, site and position**.

The next step is to consider any potential critical events. The lead surgeon will be asked to anticipate the amount of **blood loss** and, if this is more than 500 ml, cross-matched blood products should be kept ready in the theatre fridge.

Furthermore:

- Is there any **specific equipment** required, such as **imaging equipment**, and is this available?
- Are there any **critical operating steps** or potential **unexpected steps** which you want your team to prepare for?
- For the anaesthetist: are there any **patient specific concerns**?
- What is the patient's ASA grade and, again, what specific monitoring equipment or other specific support is required?

For the Scrub Team

Is the **sterility of the instruments** confirmed? Does he/she have any **concerns or issues with the required equipment**? The **surgical site infection bundle** is then covered and this requires the team to check whether:

- **prophylactic antibiotics** have been given within the last 60 minutes?
- **patient warming** is required and, if so, is it in place?
- the patient's **glycaemic control** is affected peri-operatively?
- **hair removal** is required?
- diathermy will be needed?

Venous-thromboembolism (VTE) and its prevention is an important topic across the NHS. The type of prophylaxis depends on the type and length of surgery, as well as the patient's individual risk factors.

Now, it is safe to proceed with the intended surgical intervention.

Maternity Cases – The 'Time Out'

The obstetrician should **check the placental site** on the most recent ultrasound scan to ensure there are no concerns. If the placenta is low lying, are there cross-matched blood products available in the fridge and is a cell saver required? The midwife or obstetrician can clarify if **cord blood** samples are needed. Also ask the midwife to check that the **urinary catheter** is draining and that, where relevant, the **fetal scalp electrode** has been removed. After completion of the 'Time Out' checklist, it is safe to commence the Caesarean section.

Gynaecological Surgery – The 'Sign Out'

After completion of the surgery, the Sign Out must be completed *before* any team member leaves the operating room. Confirm the **name of the procedure** has been **recorded** in the operating book. Ask the scrub nurse to confirm that the **instrument, swabs and sharps counts** are complete and correct. This is vital as retention of a swab or instrument post-operatively is totally avoidable if safety systems are in place; thus retained swabs or instruments are considered a '**Never event'**.

Ensure that you have **labelled the specimens.** Were there any **equipment problems** and does this need to be addressed? The anaesthetist needs to make sure that all the cannulas are flushed.

Finally, both the surgeon and the anaesthetist should clarify any **key concerns for the recovery** and post-operative management of the patient. Hand over appropriately to the theatre nurse who will accompany the patient to recovery, and make sure that you write any post-operative instructions on your operation note. The checklist is now complete.

Maternity Cases – The 'Sign Out'

The maternity checklist has a few additional checks to the gynaecological surgery 'Sign Out'. **Blood loss** is sometimes significant following CS and this must be escalated. Pregnant women have an increased risk of VTE and undergoing a CS adds to this risk, so ensure that **VTE prophylaxis** has been prescribed for the post-operative period. Check that the newborn **baby** has been **labelled** with a hospital name band. If required, have the **cord bloods** been taken and have the **blood gas** results been recorded?

The maternity checklist is now complete and team members are free to leave theatre.

Conclusion

Used correctly, the WHO Surgical Safety Checklist is a simple but thorough way of communicating relevant information effectively. It has already shown significant changes to morbidity and mortality rates in hospitals where the process is carried out.

Further Reading

Gawande, A.A., Thomas, E.J., Zinner, M.J., and Brennan, T.A. (1999). The incidence and nature of surgical adverse events in Colorado and Utah in 1992. *Surg.* 126: 66–75.

Haynes, A.B., Weiser, T.G., Berry, W.R. et al. (2009). A surgical safety checklist to reduce morbidy and mortality in a global population. *N. Engl. J. Med.* 360 (5): 491–499.

National Patient Safety Agency (2009). WHO Surgical Safety Checklist: A Patient Safety Update.

Weiser, T.G., Regenbogen, S.E., Thompson, K.D. et al. (2008). An estimation of the global volume of surgery; a modeling strategy based on available data. *Lancet* 372: 139–144.

World Alliance for Patient Safety (2008). *WHO Guidelines for Safe Surgery*. Geneva: World Health Organization.

3 Understanding Human Factors (Non-technical Skills) in Obstetrics and Gynaecology

Wai Yoong, Mark Ponnusamy, Roberto De Martino, and Maud Nauta

Overview

This chapter describes the rationale behind a growing need to introduce human factors (HF) or **non-technical skills (NTS)** into training schemes for healthcare professionals. Pioneered by the aviation industry, it is increasingly recognised that by focusing on specific personal qualities, attributes and skills that can be measured and trained, an individual's performance is optimised, leading to improved patient outcomes. Components of HF will be discussed to illustrate how these skills can be applied and translated to obstetrics and gynaecology. The importance of these skills for the trainee in ever-changing teams will be highlighted and tools used for integrating HF into obstetrics and gynaecology training elaborated, along with its methodological challenges.

Introduction

In this chapter, the authors outline what are referred to as **HF** or **NTS,** often erroneously considered as 'soft skills' by many professionals. Much of the pioneering work in this field was initiated by the aviation industry over 30 years ago, which resulted in the worldwide adoption of **crew resource management (CRM) training.** HF and CRM are well established as essential components in the training and assessment of aircrew. There is an impressive array of academic literature on the matter and many of the tools developed have cross-discipline applications in other professions, especially healthcare.

How to Perform Operative Procedures in Obstetrics and Gynaecology, First Edition.
Edited by Wai Yoong, Abha Govind, and Wasim Lodhi.
© 2020 John Wiley & Sons Ltd. Published 2020 by John Wiley & Sons Ltd.
Companion website: www.wiley.com/go/yoong/obgyn

Longitudinal studies in the United Kingdom have demonstrated that 50% of direct maternal deaths involve **substandard care** (Lewis 2007), with poor inter-professional teamwork along with communication problems being consistently implicated (Knight et al. 2018). The authors argue that performance of trainees can be optimised by developing HF skills, whilst simultaneously improving their technical skills.

HF in Aviation

Over the past three decades, investigations into a series of high-profile aviation accidents have uncovered that the primary causes are often not technical error or deviations from standard operating procedures, but rather the **behaviour** of the personnel operating the aircraft. Problems relating to communication, teamwork, decision-making and leadership, compounded by fatigue and stress, were all implicated in the accidents that occurred (Wieck 1990). After much research into identifying these underlying causations of accidents, the International Civil Aviation Organisation (ICAO) mandated **standardised HF and CRM training** for all professional flight crew. The airline industry is investing a large amount of time, effort and finance into providing aircrew with this compulsory annual training, with the primary aims of reducing errors and maximising operational performance.

HF in Healthcare

Echoing developments in the aviation industry, a number of high-profile cases in healthcare have shown that lack of technical skill and knowledge alone are not the explanations for adverse events. The tragic **case of Elaine Bromiley** highlighted the fact that awareness of HF was lacking in many areas of healthcare: Mrs Bromiley had been admitted for a routine surgical procedure but difficulties in intubation resulted in a prolonged period of hypoxia leading to severe brain damage and her eventual death. Three experienced senior anaesthetists attempted intubation for an extended duration of time and reflected afterwards that they should have resorted to another choice of airway management sooner: they became 'target fixated' on achieving intubation and were not aware of the passage of time. An independent review later noted that contributory factors included lack of time perception, suboptimal communication, hierarchy and the broader concept of loss of situational awareness (SA) (Harmer 2005). The Chief Medical Officer's Report in 2008 stated that perhaps Elaine Bromiley's death could have been averted if the theatre team had a better insight into '**crisis resource management**' skills (similar to the CRM domain recognised by the aviation industry) and if they had regular emergency simulation training to refine these skills.

The **National Quality Board** (a body that includes NHS England, the National Institute for Health and Care Excellence [NICE], the Care Quality Commission [CQC], Health Education England [HEE], the General Medical Council [GMC] and the Nursing and Midwifery Council [NMC]) signed a **Concordat** in 2013, supporting the National Health Service (NHS) in raising awareness and promoting HF principles and practices as well as embedding these in healthcare. The Concordat also sought to develop:

- understanding of HF in the NHS;
- inclusion of HF principles and practices in core education and training curricula for health professionals and to support ongoing professional development;
- a just, open and positive **organisational culture** that optimises human performance

and acknowledges the potential for human error at all levels and ensures a systematic approach to learning

MBRRACE-UK Maternity Reports now acknowledge the role that HF play in many underlying maternal deaths (Knight et al. 2018) and, typically, the main factor highlighted is 'the loss of situational awareness, particularly **delays in recognising the severity of the problem**'. Similarly, loss of team SA, a hierarchical management structure leading to fixation on financial targets rather than patient care, plus a catalogue of HF errors were identified by Sir Robert Francis in the public inquiry he conducted on the **Mid Staffordshire Hospital** in 2013. Each Baby Counts (RCOG 2017) analysed data from 550 term stillbirths, neonatal deaths and babies with hypoxic ischaemic encephalopathy during 2015 and the reports presented key findings and recommendations. It included a chapter on HF, stating that **loss of situational awareness, communication errors and lack of leadership** were the commonest contributory factors accounting for 44, 45 and 22% of cases respectively. The RCOG has also provided a toolkit, audio-visual resources and teaching material on understanding and implementing aspects of HF on the labour ward based on this report (www.rcog.org.uk/globalassets/documents/guidelines/research--audit/rcog-each-baby-counts-report.pdf).

Defining HF

HF encompasses a range of cognitive and social elements which complement knowledge and technical skills to enable maximal performance. Specific nomenclature has been developed applicable to a particular profession or role, and listed below is the widely accepted classification which divides HF into five broad areas:

1 communication
2 situational awareness
3 problem-solving and decision-making
4 leadership and team-working
5 workload management.

The aviation industry has established a set of behavioural markers as an aid for aircrew to measure the effectiveness of their HF skills as applied to their role and these are listed in Table 3.1.

Communication Skills

Good communication underpins and is a ubiquitous prerequisite for all of the skills within the HF framework. However, the ability to communicate well is often overlooked and taken for granted during training; the communication skills demanded of trainees in potential stressful adverse events are rarely practised other than in simulated environments (Boxes 3.1 and 3.2).

Situational Awareness (SA)

The definition of SA as 'the perception of elements in the environment within a volume of time and space, the comprehension of their meaning, and the projection of their status in the near future' is well established across multiple task domains (Endsley 1995). This can be seen as having application in achieving **immediate tactical objectives** in complex environments; having SA also helps to develop understanding and recognition of the significance of the order of events. The aviation, military and nuclear industries, as well as traditional occupational psychologists, have made meaningful contributions to the understanding of the concept.

Pilots often use the **acronym:**

N	notice
U	understand
T	think
A	ahead

to help simplify the concept of SA.

Table 3.1 Non-technical standards.

Non-Technical Skills	
	Observable actions
Communication skills	• Know precisely what, how much and who they need to communicate with. • Ensure the recipient is prepared and able to receive and retain the information. • Convey information clearly and accurately. • Confirm the recipient has the correct understanding. • Use appropriate non-verbal communication. • Are open and receptive to other people's views.
Situational awareness	Are aware of what the team are doing and its goals. Keep track of time and resources. Recognise what is likely to happen, anticipate, plan and stay ahead of the game. Are aware of the team's interactions with the environment. Are aware of the condition of the people involved, including other healthcare workers besides the patients. Identify threats to the health and safety of the patient and the team.
Problem-solving and decision-making	Identify and analyse why errors occur. Do not jump to conclusions or make assumptions. Seek accurate and adequate information from appropriate resources. Use and agree an effective decision-making process. Consider risks but do not take avoidable risks.
Leadership and team-working	Be clear on the team's objectives and members' roles. Use initiative, give direction and take responsibility when required. Be honest. Give and receive criticism and praise well, and admit mistakes. Demonstrate respect, empathy and tolerance for other people. Involve others in planning and share activities fairly. Be friendly, enthusiastic, motivating and considerate to the team.

In complex scenarios, cognitive overload can overwhelm the capability of a novice, so they are less able to observe, process and integrate information efficiently.

In contrast, experienced decision-makers assess and interpret the current situation and select an appropriate action based on conceptual patterns stored in their long-term

Box 3.1 Herald of Free Enterprise Incident

The maritime disaster of the capsizing of the Herald of Free Enterprise in 1987, resulting in the deaths of 193 passengers and crew, was the worst peace-time maritime disaster in living memory. After leaving port, the ship's bow doors were not closed and within 90 seconds of leaving Dover harbour, water began entering the car deck. The resulting free surface effect of water flowing unopposed across the large area of car deck destroyed the ship's stability; after listing to port (i.e. tilting to the left side) the ship capsized within 90 seconds. A subsequent enquiry found that poor communication between personnel as well as a failure of confirmation of safety procedures led to one member of crew failing to check the bow doors were closed, and the captain leaving port assuming the bow doors were closed. Following this adverse event, a system of compulsory communication of positive system checks was instituted, as well as lights displaying the state of the bow doors on the bridge. This illustrates how poor communication can impact on a team's operational ability during routine procedures, as well as in stressful situations; the concept of compulsory communication of essential information is used routinely in the World Health Organization (WHO) theatre checklist before and after completing an operation. Studies of adverse events in surgery (Wilson 1999) and obstetrics (Guise and Segel 2008) have identified communication as the causal factor in approximately half the errors made. A joint commission into the study of errors in obstetric care also concluded that failure of team work and communication were the cause of 70% of adverse events (Bahl et al. 2010), illustrating a learning and training need which can be addressed through training tools such as simulation. There is a great deal of literature on communication skills and it should be emphasised that training and assessment of communication skills is central to developing HF awareness and practice.

Box 3.2 Retained Swab after Surgery

A 45 year-old lady with heavy periods underwent vaginal myomectomy via Duhrssen's incision (Duhrssen 1890) for a 4 cm submucous fibroid located close to the cervix. Due to the venous ooze from the base, the inflated balloon of a Foley's catheter was used to tamponade the base and vaginal pack was left in situ near the site of the fibroid excision. This was clearly documented in the notes with specific instructions for removal the following day. The patient was reviewed by the on call registrar the next morning and was discharged after nursing staff reported that the pack and Foley's catheter had been removed. The patient was readmitted five days later with a foul vaginal discharge and the retained pack was found in the vagina and promptly removed.

Root cause analysis showed significant miscommunication between the night shift agency nurse who had incorrectly reported that the vaginal pack had been removed (she had confused the term 'pack' with 'pad' and had meant that the patient's sanitary pad had been removed) and the duty registrar (who had not verified the nurse's statement).

Apart from poor communication, non-regular staff and unusual/emergency operations are common contributory factors in cases of retained swabs.

Since the occurrence of this Serious Untoward Incident (SUI), colour-coded wristbands as well as checklists have been introduced to record insertion and removal of vaginal packs following surgery.

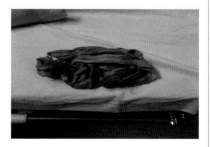

Box 3.3   Situational Awareness

Notice (Perception): The patient is bleeding. The more sutures I put in, the more she bleeds.
Understand (Comprehension): She is developing coagulopathy (DIC).
Think Ahead (Projection): I won't put in any more sutures. Let's correct the coagulopathy and transfer her to ITU. Let me call for senior help.

memory as a mental model (Box 3.3). Having inadequate SA has been identified as one of the primary factors in adverse events attributed to human error (Merket et al. 1997).

As illustrated in the **Elaine Bromiley case** discussed earlier, poor SA can occur across a team as well as within an individual. Team SA can be defined as 'the degree to which every team member possesses the SA required for his or her responsibilities' (Endsley 1995). These attributes contribute to the success of a team and this is facilitated by team members sharing similar mental models. **Dysfunctional team working,** as identified by Dr William Kirkup in the Kirkup Report of Morecombe Bay Maternity Services (Kirkup 2015), can lead to divergent objectives and inconsistent mental models.

Problem-Solving and Decision-Making

Decision-making is a cognitive process resulting in the selection of a course of action amongst several alternatives to provide the best outcome, with every decision-making process ideally producing a final choice (Reason 2000).

Professor Daniel Kahneman of Princeton University (Kahneman 2011) postulated that our thinking brain is engaged in a continual struggle between **intuition** (System 1) and **logic** (System 2). System 1 is fast, automatic, emotional and unconscious, whilst System 2 is slow, effortful, logical and conscious. These systems drive our decision-making processes and can be simplified into two basic cognitive decision-making models: the **naturalistic and analytical models**. Furthermore, we sometimes utilise a third model known as '**rule-based**' decision-making which is especially useful in complex or time-pressured situations. A typical example would be the 'Can't intubate, can't ventilate' protocol where an established set of rules lead the decision-maker rapidly through a decision tree that ultimately leads to a tracheostomy. In rule-based decision-making, experts have done the thinking and produced a set of rules that can be followed by the decision-maker to achieve the required outcome for pre-set circumstances in time-critical situations.

Naturalistic decision-making (System 1) uses less cognitive processing and can be likened to intuition. Although highly skilled and trained professionals ('experts') like to believe that they make decisions using System 2, Klein et al. (1986) have shown that experts can make fast and intuitive decisions even when under time pressure using a combination of experience, training and 'heuristics' or cognitive shortcuts.

Analytical decision-making (System 2) is a structured process that takes time and cognitive effort and uses the 'thinking' brain. It is well suited to unexpected, unusual or complex situations where the decision-maker has limited previous experience.

Each of these decision-making processes have their pros and cons.

Naturalistic decision-making uses 'pattern recognition', experience and previous training and is therefore fast, thereby freeing up cognitive capacity for other tasks. It is, however, vulnerable to heuristic bias, such as **anchoring** (relying too heavily on one piece of information) or **availability** (giving weight to examples that we easily recall) and short cuts such as **satisficing** (settling on an acceptable solution but not necessarily the optimal one).

Analytical decision-making uses structure and encourages options generation and a review process. It is ideal for unusual or complex situations when decisions need to be made by less experienced individuals. It is, however, time consuming and vulnerable to interruptions and distractions and can result in poor outcomes due to **confirmation bias** (giving weight to evidence that confirms the original model instead of the differential evidence).

Military aviation offers its aviators a model known as **RAPDAR** which provides the necessary structure for analytical decision-making under time constraints (Table 3.2).

Leadership and Teamwork

Most day-to-day tasks in Obstetrics and Gynaecology are performed by small teams, usually led by consultants, senior trainees or senior midwives. This issue of clinical leadership has been long debated and there are two generalised opinions.

A good leader is essential in order for a team to be effective.

Although a leader is required, it may not be the most important factor in a team's success.

A **good team leader** clearly communicates the team's objectives and members' roles, uses initiative, takes responsibility and also demonstrates respect, empathy and tolerance. Where a team is disorganised and lacks clear objectives, an influential figure who provides directional control and authority is necessary. Conversely, if members already have defined roles, are motivated, communicate well and are organised, the team will function effectively irrespective of a leader. The role of the leader then changes from that of an autocrat to one of **final decision-maker** and **general organisational facilitator.** This is what tends to occur in most effective clinical teams and is the model preferred in healthcare.

Teamwork training has been shown to be successful in reducing technical errors and is an essential component of any HF programme. With the implementation of the **European Working Time Directive** (EWTD), trainees in obstetrics and gynaecology will now work a maximum of 48 hour per week (approximately half that of their

Table 3.2   RAPDAR.

Recognise	Identify significant factors or events, continual monitoring and cross referencing to 'the norm' is required.
Analyse	Likely effects of the recognised events or factors and project possible action.
Prioritise	Multiple events, factors or analyses.
Decide	Make your decision.
Act	Implement your decision.
Review	Review the effects and success of your actions.

predecessors), thus limiting their clinical exposure to surgical procedures as well as to potentially difficult scenarios involving teams. Furthermore, many trainees now work on **shift patterns** with a varied composition of staff, where they remain individually accountable for their professional conduct and care (GMC 2006). This is analogous to the aviation industry which often works with ever changing team members and sometimes in an unfamiliar environment. For this process to remain safe and effective mandates the acquisition of team skill sets which include development of a shallow authority gradient and sharing mental models through briefings and communication tools (such as **SBAR**).

Workload Management

Workload management encompasses the ability to manage time efficiently, prioritise, acknowledge limits and ensure the completion of tasks with the available resources. The 6 Ps (Proper Planning and Preparation Prevents Poor Performance) is an old axiom that reminds us of the pivotal role of organisation in workload management, as does the saying 'fail to prepare, prepare to fail'. Workload management is focused around the central concepts of **planning, prioritisation and predicting** all possible eventualities. Good workload management mitigates the need for anxiety, minimises distractions and enables the mind to function at full capacity as well as to remain calm under pressure. This is a skill that busy trainees in obstetrics and gynaecology will require during on-call, theatre sessions and clinics.

Examples of Implementation of HF in Training Curriculum

There are two major examples where NTS training and assessment has been implemented in healthcare in the United Kingdom. **NOTSS** (Non-Technical Skills for Surgeons) was created to provide a tool to observe and rate the behavioural aspects of performance of surgeons in the operating theatre in a structured manner. This was developed from and shared many tools with Anaesthetists Non-Technical Skills (**ANTS**) and Scottish studies on surgical competence and professionalism where certain cognitive and interpersonal skills were identified as being relevant for surgeons to operate reliably and safely (Yule et al. 2008). Table 3.3 shows a completed example of NOTSS rating form from a trainee's operation.

Regional workshops on NTS have also been started by deaneries who train facilitators who can then implement local training, often incorporating serious incident reports into scenario designs in order to identify learning points.

Conclusion

HF, often referred to as CRM, is an established scientific discipline used in many other safety critical industries. HF underpins current patient safety and quality improvement science, offering an integrated, evidenced and coherent approach to patient safety, quality improvement and clinical excellence.

The principles and practices of HF focus on optimising human performance through better understanding the behaviour of individuals, their interactions with each other and with their environment. By acknowledging human limitations, it offers ways to minimise and mitigate human frailties, so reducing medical error and its consequences. The system-wide adoption of these concepts offers a unique opportunity to support cultural change and empower the NHS to put patient safety and clinical excellence at its heart.

Hospital .... Trainer name .... Date ....

Trainee name .... Operation ....

Category	Category rating*	Element	Element rating*	Feedback on performance and debriefing notes
Situation awareness		Gathering information		
		Understanding information		
		Projecting and anticipating future state		
Decision-making		Considering options		
		Selecting and communicating option		
		Implementing and reviewing decisions		
Communication and teamwork		Exchanging information		
		Establishing a shared understanding		
		Coordinating team activities		
Leadership		Setting and maintaining standards		
		Supporting others		
		Coping with pressure		

* **1** Poor; **2** Marginal; **3** Acceptable; **4** Good; **NA** Not applicable

1 Poor	Performance endangered or potentially endangered patient safety; serious remediation is required
2 Marginal	Performance indicated cause for concern; considerable improvement is needed
3 Acceptable	Performance was of a satisfactory standard but could be improved
4 Good	Performance was of a consistently high standard, enhancing patient safety; it could be used as a positive example for others
NA	Not applicable

Figure 3.1 NOTSS tool using behavioural markers to assess SA. *Source*: Crossley et al. 2011.

Further Reading

Bahl, R., Murphy, D.J., and Strachan, B. (2010). Non-technical skills for obstetricians conducting forceps and vacuum deliveries: qualitative analysis by interviews and video recordings. *Eur. J. Obstet. Gynecol. Reprod. Biol.* 150 (2): 147–151.

Crossley, J.G.M., Marriott, J., Purdie, H., and Beard, J.D. (2011). Prospective observational study to evaluate NOTSS (Non-Technical Skills for Surgeons) for assessing trainees' non-technical performance in the operating theatre. *Br. J. Surg.* 98 (7): 1010–1020.

Duhrssen, A. (1890). Uber den Werth der tiefen Cervix-und Scheiden-Damm-Einschnitte in der Geburtshulfe. *Arch. Gynaek.* 37: 27–66.

Endsley, M.R. (1995). Toward a theory of situation awareness in dynamic systems. *Hum. Factors* 37 (1): 32–64.

Francis, R. (2013). Report on The Mid Staffordshire NHS Foundation Trust Inquiry. London: The Stationary Office. HC 947. 6 February 2013.

General Medical Council (2006). Good Medical Practice. Working with Colleagues/Working in Teams. Paragraphs 41–42. London: GMC.

Guise, J.M. and Segel, S. (2008). Teamwork in obstetric critical care. *Best Pract. Res. Clin. Obstet. Gynaecol.* 22: 937–951.

Harmer, M. (2005). Independent Review on the care given to Mrs Elaine Bromiley on 29 March 2005. http://www.chfg.org/wpcontent/uploads/ElaineBromileyAnonymousReport.pdf

Human Factors in Healthcare (2013). A Concordat from the National Quality Board. https://www.england.nhs.uk/wp-content/uploads/2013/11/nqb-hum-fact-concord.pdf.

Kahneman, D. (2011). *Thinking Fast and Slow*. London: Penguin Books Ltd.

Kirkup, W. (2015). The Report of the Morecambe Bay Investigation March 2015. https://assets.publishing.service.gov.uk/government/uploads/system/uploads/attachment_data/file/408480/47487_MBI_Accessible_v0.1.pdf.

Klein, G.A., Calderwood, R., and Clinton-Cirocco, A. (1986). Rapid decision making on the fireground. *Journal of Cognitive Engineering and Decision Making* 4 (3): 186–209.

Knight, M., Bunch, K., Tuffnell, D., et al. (eds) on behalf of MBRRACE-UK (2018). Saving Lives, Improving Mothers' Care - Lessons Learned to Inform Maternity Care from the UK and Ireland Confidential Enquiries into Maternal Deaths and Morbidity 2014–16. Oxford: National Perinatal Epidemiology Unit, University of Oxford.

Lewis, G. (ed.) (2007). The Confidential Enquiry into Maternal and Child Health (CEMACH). Saving Mothers' Lives: Reviewing Maternal Deaths to Make Motherhood Safer—2003–2005. The Seventh Report on Confidential Enq uiries into Maternal Deaths in the United Kingdom. London, United Kingdom: Confidential Enquiry into Maternal and Child Health.

Merket, D.C., Bergondy, N., and Cuevas-Mesa, H. (1997). Making sense out of teamwork errors in complex environments. Abstract presented at the 18th Annual Industrial/Organizational-Organizational Behavior Graduate Student Conference, Ranaoke, VA.

RCOG (2017). Each Baby Counts. www.rcog.org.uk/en/guidelines-research-services/audit-quality-improvement/each-baby-counts/implementation/improving-human-factors/video-briefing.

Reason, J. (2000). Human error: models and management. *West. J. Med.* 172 (6): 393–396.

Wieck, K. (1990). The vulnerable system: an analysis of the Tenerife air disaster. *J. Manag.* 16: 571–593.

Wilson, J. (1999). A practical guide to risk management in surgery; developing and planning. Healthcare risk resources international. Royal College of Surgeons Symposium.

Yule, S., Flin, R., Paterson-Brown, S. et al. (2008). Surgeon's non-technical skills in the operating room reliability testing of the NOTSS behaviour rating system. *World J. Surg.* 32: 548–556.

4 Surgical Instruments

Christina Neophytou, Rajvinder Khasriya, and Wai Yoong

Video Duration | 10 mins 37 secs

Overview

It is important that trainees learn the names and functions of basic surgical instruments. Currently there are very few courses that formally teach these. This chapter aims to help you recognise the **eponymous instruments** commonly used in obstetric and gynaecological procedures and learn their functions and indications of use.

Introduction

A good basic comprehension of the tools and understanding why they are perfectly crafted for their use will allow you to develop as a surgeon. It will enable you to confidently ask for the right instrument in the case of an unfamiliar scenario.

We have organised this chapter to include the **commonly used** instruments that you will encounter during your practice depending on their function.

Categorising instruments according to the surgical operations they are often used in facilitates learning and memorisation of the eponymous names. Tables 4.1–4.3 list the set of instruments used in: (i) Caesarean section; (ii) laparotomy/total abdominal hysterectomy; and (iii) vaginal hysterectomy.

Surgical Scalpel

Surgical scalpels are made up of two parts: a blade and a handle (Figure 4.1). The handles are reusable, whilst the blades are disposable. The **handle** is also known as a 'B.P handle', after the **Bard-Parker** Company. The handles come in different shapes: the #3 and #4 handles are flat whilst the #7 handle resembles a long writing pen, rounded at the front and flat at the back. A #4 handle is larger than a #3 handle. Fully disposable scalpels are also available. They usually have a plastic handle with an extensible blade and are for single use only.

Needle Holders

Needle holders (Figures 4.2a and b) have a **ratchet mechanism** that **locks** the needle in place. This allows the user to manoeuvre

How to Perform Operative Procedures in Obstetrics and Gynaecology, First Edition.
Edited by Wai Yoong, Abha Govind, and Wasim Lodhi.
© 2020 John Wiley & Sons Ltd. Published 2020 by John Wiley & Sons Ltd.
Companion website: www.wiley.com/go/yoong/obgyn

Table 4.1 Surgical instrument set for Caesarean section.

- Mayo scissors 14.5 cm TC Straight
- Mayo scissors 14.5 cm TC Curved
- Mayo-Hegar needle holder 16 cm TC
- Heaney needle holder 21 cm TC 01
- Bard-Parker scalpel handle #4
- Blades for scalpel handle #4
- Stille forceps 20 cm
- Rampley or Bonney dissecting forceps 16 cm
- Lane forceps 1 : 2 18 cm
- Kelly forceps 14 cm Straight
- Kelly forceps 14 cm Curved
- Crile forceps 1 : 2 14 cm
- Allis tissue forceps 4 : 5 19 cm
- Backhaus towel forceps 11 cm
- Doyen retractor 50 × 85 mm 25 cm
- Kelly retractor 65 × 50 mm 26 cm
- Rampley sponge forceps 25 cm
- Diathermy forceps, lead and quiver
- Green-Armytage haemostatic clamp

Table 4.2 Surgical instrument set for laparotomy/total abdominal hysterectomy.

- Mayo-Hegar needle holders
- Scissors: 1 Suture cutting, 1 Mayo curved 7 1/2, 1 Mayo straight 7 1/2
- Poole sucker
- Diathermy forceps
- Diathermy lead
- Diathermy quiver
- Bozemann packing forceps
- Bonney myomectomy screw
- Gwilliams, Rogers or Maingot hysterectomy clamps
- Teale vulsellum
- Rampley sponge forceps
- Backhaus towel clip
- Dissecting forceps: Ramsey or Bonney toothed and non-toothed forceps
- Artery forceps: Spencer-Wells, Kocher straight/curved and Dunhill forceps
- Babcock tissue forceps
- Tissue forceps: Allis, Littlewood
- Bard-Parker knife handle
- Retractors: Landon, Morris, Deaver, Langenbeck, and Balfour

the needle through various tissues in different planes. It is advised that the needle holder is closed on the first or second ratchet as holding the needle too tightly may break or bend the needle. The jaws of the needle holders are textured and short when compared to the handles in order to maintain a good grip on the needle. They can sometimes be confused with Spencer-Wells tissue forceps, which have longer and thinner jaws. The length of the needle holder depends on the access required. A haemostatic suture to be placed deep in the pelvis requires a **long-handled** needle holder, whilst a skin suture can be inserted using a **shorter** needle **holder**.

Scissors

Scissors are broadly classified into **dissecting or suture cutting** scissors. Dissecting (or tissue cutting) scissors such as Mayo scissors are usually curved and heavy and are used to cut through tough scar tissue (Figure 4.3). **McIndoe** dissecting scissors (Figure 4.4) are used for finer dissection. They are often inserted with the blades closed and then gently opened to bluntly dissect through anatomical planes. Suture scissors are straight and lighter.

Forceps

Forceps are generally used to **grasp** tissue. This instrument is usually held between thumb and forefinger in a pincer grip

Table 4.3 Gynaecological instrument set for vaginal hysterectomy.

- Auvard vaginal speculum
- Sims vaginal speculum
- Rampley sponge forceps
- Polyp forceps
- Single-toothed tenaculum
- Teale vulsellum
- Uterine sound
- Hegar dilators
- Bard-Parker blade handle
- 2 × small Spencer-Wells artery forceps
- Small artery forceps
- Uterine curettes
- Medium-toothed dissecting forceps
- Mayo suture scissors
- Mayo-Hegar needle holders
- Gwilliams, Rogers or Maingot hysterectomy clamps
- Lone Star retractor
- Angled or Breisky retractor

(a)

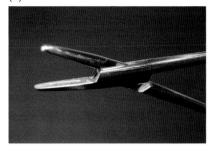

(b)

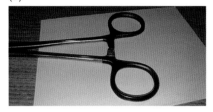

Figure 4.2   (a) Needle holder and (b) ratchet mechanism.

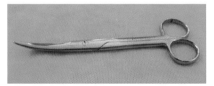

Figure 4.3   Mayo scissors.

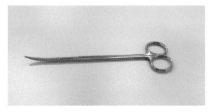

Figure 4.4   McIndoe scissors.

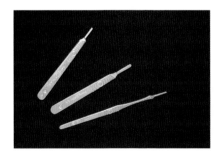

Figure 4.1   Surgical scalpel handles #3, #4, and #7 (left to right).

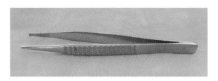

Figure 4.5   Ramsey toothed forceps.

(usually with the **left hand** if you are right-handed) to manipulate the needle and grasp tissue **edges** when suturing. They can be **toothed** or **non-toothed**, fine or robust and can vary in their length.

Ramsey toothed forceps (Figure 4.5) are excellent for traction and securely gripping tissue. Caution should be taken when using

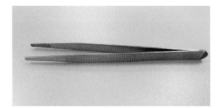

Figure 4.6 Ramsey non-toothed forceps.

toothed forceps as they can be **traumatic** to tissues. Ramsey non-toothed forceps (Figure 4.6) is therefore the preferred type of forceps to minimise trauma when used inside the **peritoneal cavity.** Fine, toothed forceps are usually used for **picking up skin edges** during skin closure.

Tissue Holding Forceps

These are **ringed** instruments that are used for **grasping** and **retracting** tissues and are **ratcheted.**

Littlewood forceps (Figure 4.7) are commonly found on the Caesarean section tray, where they are used to **hold the rectus sheath** to aid dissection and to identify edges when suturing the sheath. As Littlewood forceps have sharp teeth, they should not be used within the peritoneal cavity.

Lane forceps (Figure 4.8) have **heavy blades** and fenestrations (an opening in the blades) and the tip has interlocking teeth that will hold and grasp any tissue. They are suitable for holding tissue such as a myoma.

Allis forceps (Figure 4.9) have **serrated jaws** and small **hinged teeth.** They are used to hold and retract **subcuticular** tissue. They can be used to hold **soft tissues** for long periods. These are used in many procedures in obstetrics and gynaecology, such as holding the torn ends of the **external anal sphincter** after a

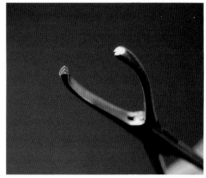

Figure 4.7 Littlewood tissue forceps.

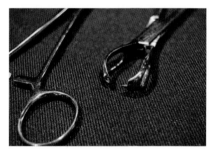

Figure 4.8 Lane tissue forceps.

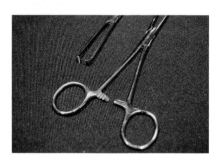

Figure 4.9 Allis tissue forceps.

third-degree tear or securing vaginal walls during **vaginal surgery.**

Green-Armytage haemostatic forceps (Figure 4.10) are flat broad instruments used to hold the incised uterine edges at **Caesarean section** prior to closing the incision. Four are commonly used; one on each side of the uterine incision angle. They

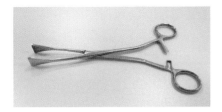

Figure 4.10   Green-Armytage haemostatic forceps.

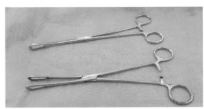

Figure 4.12   Rampley sponge forceps.

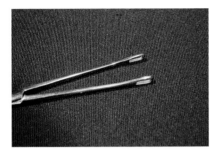

Figure 4.11   Polyp forceps.

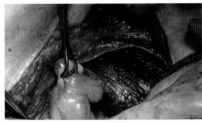

Figure 4.13   Babcock tissue forceps holding the appendix.

have **triangulated tips** which are serrated at the inner edge. This allows **large uterine sinuses** to be **compressed** to curb bleeding. They could also be used to grasp the cervix to stop bleeding of a tear.

Polyp and **Rampley sponge forceps** do not have sharp hooks or teeth but small **transverse grooves**. Polyp forceps (Figure 4.11) are used to firmly grasp uterine **polyps** and **avulse** them at polypectomy. They can also be used to retrieve foreign objects such as a lost **intra-uterine coil or** for **grasping the cervix** in the presence of any cervical trauma or to apply pressure to a bleeding vessel.

A swab on a stick is provided by **wrapping** a **gauze** swab around the Rampley sponge forceps (Figure 4.12). This is useful for 'prepping' the **skin**, swabbing the **paracolic gutters** at Caesarean section and for gently **manipulating bowel.**

Babcock forceps (Figure 4.13) have **atraumatic loop tips** and a blunt broad

base. They are useful in holding **delicate or damaged tissue** such as **fallopian tubes, ovary, ureters, bowel and appendix.**

Retractors

Retractors assist surgery by **improving** the surgical **field of view.** They are used to **hold back** the **abdominal** or **vaginal walls** and/or viscus. They can be **hand-held** or **self-retaining**. It is worth noting that if used for long periods of time, self-retaining retractors can cause bruising or nerve compression.

Doyen retractors (Figure 4.14) are used at Caesarean section to retract the bladder away from the incision site and protect it against potential injury when suturing. They are usually removed prior to delivery of the baby and reinserted after delivery to allow a good view of the lower edge of the uterine incisions.

Langenbeck retractors (Figure 4.15) are light, **L-shaped** retractors with a flat blade.

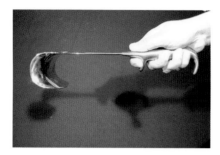

Figure 4.14   Doyen retractor.

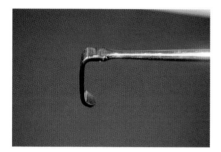

Figure 4.15   Langenbeck retractor.

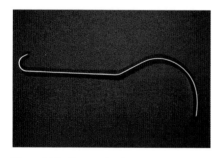

Figure 4.16   Deaver retractor.

They are used to **retract skin** during closure of the rectus sheath at Caesarean section and laparotomy. They are also used in vaginal surgery to **retract** the **vaginal walls.**

Deaver retractor (Figure 4.16) is a **manual** retractor. It comes in various sizes and is used in abdominal operations to **retract** the **viscera**. The curving C-shape allows the Deaver to follow the curve of the

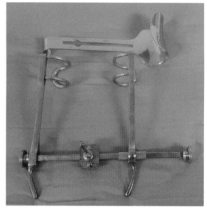

Figure 4.17   Balfour self-retaining retractor.

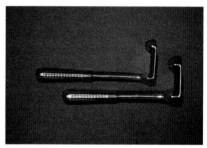

Figure 4.18   Morris retractors (side view).

anterior abdominal wall and allow **retraction of deep** structures.

A **Balfour** retractor (Figure 4.17) is **self-retaining** and used for different types of **abdominal** surgery, including total abdominal **hysterectomy.** There is a single **central wide curved blade** to hold back the bladder and small **lateral blades** which hold apart the abdominal wound. This retractor is often used to hold the bowel back after packing with large swabs for exposure of the pelvic organs. The **Morris** retractor (Figure 4.18) is a **smaller hand-held** retractor, commonly used to retract wound edges at opening and closing of the abdomen.

Haemostatic Clamps and Artery Forceps

Haemostatic clamps such as **Gwilliams** and **Rogers** (Figure 4.19), are used on vascular pedicles during **abdominal** or **vaginal hysterectomy.** They are sturdy and have atraumatic jaws to minimise tissue trauma. They have **longitudinal grooves** that prevent inadvertent slippage of vessels.

Spencer-Wells artery forceps (Figure 4.20) are commonly used for **grasping bleeding tissues** and bluntly dissecting tissues along normal anatomical planes. They have rigid teeth that improve compression and grip of tissue. They are used in pairs for **clamping** a section of the **umbilical cord** prior to dividing and can also be used as **'clips'** on stay sutures.

Kocher forceps (Figure 4.21) have serrated blades and interlocking teeth at the tips. They are also used for **blunt dissection** and for holding gauze pellets or **pledgets**.

Dunhill artery forceps (Figure 4.22) are small, curved instruments for grasping bleeding tissues or **small vessels** prior to ligation or cauterisation. They are **finer** than Spencer-Wells forceps and can also be used as 'clips' on stay sutures.

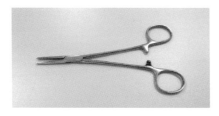

Figure 4.20   Spencer-Wells artery forceps.

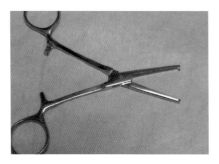

Figure 4.21   Kocher artery forceps.

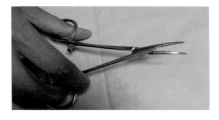

Figure 4.22   Dunhill artery forceps.

(a)

(b)

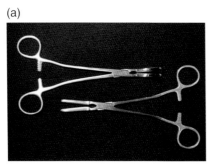

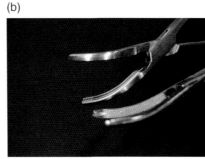

Figure 4.19   (a) Rogers straight and curved clamps and (b) Rogers vs Maingot clamps.

Other Miscellaneous Instruments

Myoma screw (Figure 4.23) is used at open myomectomy. It is applied in a **clockwise** motion into a fibroid to provide good leverage and traction.

Sims speculum (Figure 4.24) is one of the most commonly used and ubiquitous instruments in our speciality. It is used for inspecting the vagina and cervix or for manually **retracting the posterior vaginal wall,** in order to allow access for vaginal surgery.

Auvard speculum (Figure 4.25) has similar function to Sims but has a **weight attached** to the end of the handle in order to facilitate **self-retraction.**

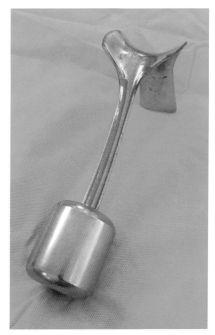

Figure 4.25 Auvard speculum.

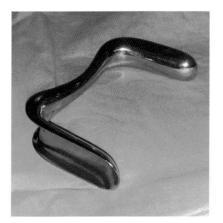

Figure 4.23 Myoma screw.

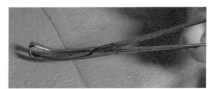

Figure 4.26 Vulsellum forceps.

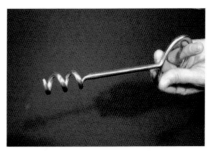

Figure 4.24 Sims speculum.

Vulsellum forceps (Figure 4.26) are used to grasp the **cervical lips** or to provide counter resistance when introducing instruments such as **dilators** or **hysteroscopes.** They have a **pelvic curve** and can be single, double or multiple **toothed.**

A **uterine sound** (Figure 4.27) is used to **measure the length** of the uterine cavity and cervical canal and to ascertain if the uterus is anteverted or retroverted. In order to minimise the risk of uterine perforation, it is advised that the sound is used with

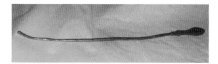

Figure 4.27 Uterine sound.

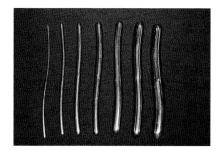

Figure 4.28 A set of Hegar dilators.

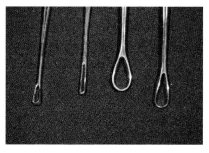

Figure 4.29 Sharp and blunt curettes.

caution and that it is guarded using the index finger at the time of insertion.

Hegar dilators (Figure 4.28) are **double-ended** smooth metallic dilators used to **dilate** the **cervix** in order to introduce other instruments such as a hysteroscope or curette.

Uterine curettes (Figure 4.29) come in different sizes and the cervix may **require dilatation** prior to their use. They are used for **endometrial sampling** in cases of abnormal bleeding and for curettage after evacuation of the uterus to **remove** retained **products of conception.**

Conclusion

This chapter has taken you through the main surgical instruments that you are likely to encounter during your career in obstetrics and gynaecology. We acknowledge that this list is not exhaustive but hope it has provided you with the solid foundation required prior to operating. We recommend that you complement your learning by spending some time with an experienced (and patient) senior scrub nurse to revise the names and functions of the instruments described above.

5 Surgical Positioning

Ciara MacKenzie, Rosalind Aughwane, Wasim Lodhi, and Wai Yoong

Video Duration | 1 min 57 secs

Overview

Surgical positioning is a subject that is not formally taught to trainees but is very important as it allows optimal access to the surgical site. The authors discuss lithotomy, Trendelenburg and Lloyd-Davies, the three most commonly used surgical positions in obstetrics and gynaecology.

Introduction

Optimal surgical positioning is imperative for good surgical access, whilst incorrect positioning can lead to haemodynamic instability, impaired ventilation and musculoskeletal injury in patients. Different positions are necessary for different surgical procedures and it is important to know not only the correct position but the advantages and disadvantages of that used. The three most commonly used surgical positions in obstetrics and gynaecology are **Lithotomy, Trendelenburg and Lloyd-Davies.** In most instances the patient will be in theatre under spinal or general anaesthesia. Before commencing any movement, the anaesthetist must be informed and often movements will only be under their specific direction. It is important to always consider health and safety and the need to avoid injury to staff when positioning patients, particularly those patients who

are obese or pregnant. In most instances a minimum of five people will be necessary to safely position a patient – the anaesthetist at the head and two people on either side of the patient. A practical guide to positioning patients is available on the accompanying DVD.

Lithotomy Position

Lithotomy position (Figure 5.1) is one of the most commonly used positions in obstetrics and gynaecology. It is used in childbirth, instrumental delivery, perineal, vaginal and urological surgery. Lithotomy position is defined as **supine position** of the body with the **legs separated, flexed and supported in raised stirrups.**

The patient starts in the supine position and is then moved down the table until the buttocks lie just beyond the edge of the lower table break. As you can see in the photos the bottom end of the table has

---

How to Perform Operative Procedures in Obstetrics and Gynaecology, First Edition.
Edited by Wai Yoong, Abha Govind, and Wasim Lodhi.
© 2020 John Wiley & Sons Ltd. Published 2020 by John Wiley & Sons Ltd.
Companion website: www.wiley.com/go/yoong/obgyn

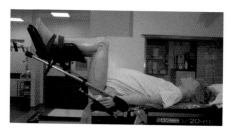

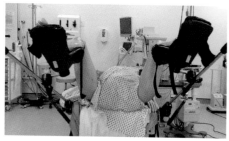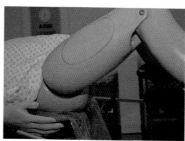

Figure 5.1 Lithotomy position.

been removed at the break. If the buttocks are not positioned just beyond the table break it will be difficult to operate and insert instruments such as the Sims speculum correctly. However, if the buttocks are too far beyond the table break they will overhang and there is a risk of the patient slipping. Once the buttocks are positioned optimally, both legs are elevated simultaneously and placed in **support boots.** This simultaneous movement helps to avoid dislocation of the hip joint, minimises risks to the other extremity, helps avoid rotational stress on the lumbar spine and maintains limbs in a symmetrical arrangement. The angle of flexion and external rotation will depend on the procedure being performed and can be adjusted using the handles at the end of the support boots.

Trendelenburg Position

Trendelenburg position (Figure 5.2) is commonly used in laparoscopic surgery and open abdominal surgery. It was initially

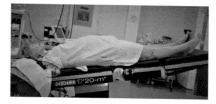

Figure 5.2 Trendelenburg position.

described as the torso supine with the legs upon the shoulders of an assistant; however, the term is now often used to describe any **head-down position – classically a 45° head-down tilt.** This position aids the surgeon's view by using **gravity** to move abdominal viscera superiorly; however, this can severely limit diaphragmatic movement, increase ventilation/perfusion mismatch and raise intracranial pressure. The patient starts in the supine position and then the table is gradually tilted head-down. It is important to always check the maximum angle of tilt with the anaesthetist before commencing any movement. The angle of tilt may be adjusted intraoperatively if there are anaesthetic concerns such as ventilation difficulties or to benefit the surgeon's view if the patient is anaesthetically stable.

Lloyd Davies Position

Lloyd Davies position (Figure 5.3) is used in pelvic and rectal surgery where access is required from both abdominal and perineal aspects. It is also known as Trendelenburg position with legs apart or head-down lithotomy. It is defined as **supine position of the body with hips flexed at 15° as the basic angle and a 30° head-down tilt.** The key difference between lithotomy and Lloyd-Davies is the degree of hip and knee flexion. The patient is moved into lithotomy position as previously described. The hips

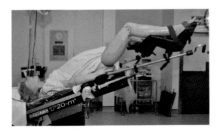

Figure 5.3   Lloyd Davies position.

should be flexed at 15°. Once the legs are secured, the table is gradually tilted head-down to 30°. As with the Trendelenburg position the exact angle of tilt is usually a compromise between anaesthetic and surgical demands. The advantage of this position is **fewer neuropathological side-effects** compared to the lithotomy position where the hips are almost fully flexed.

6 Sutures and Needles

Rosalind Aughwane, Ciara MacKenzie, Wasim Lodhi, and Wai Yoong

Video Duration | 5 mins 29 secs

Overview

A basic understanding of sutures, suture material and needles must be gained so that the optimal choice can be made for any given procedure.

Introduction

It is very important to know the different types of needles and sutures available and the relative advantages and disadvantages of those used. Although the nomenclature and vast array available may seem overwhelming, a basic understanding must be gained so that the optimal choice of needle and suture is made for any given procedure. A practical guide to sutures and needles is available in the accompanying instructional DVD.

Needles

Needles are designed to carry suture material through tissue with the minimal amount of trauma. Surgical needles have three basic components – the **attachment point, the body and the point.**

The Attachment

The majority of sutures used have an appropriate needle attached. These so-called swaged needles are convenient and minimise tissue trauma (Figure 6.1). They are subdivided into standard needle attachment and removable needle attachments which, as the name suggests, can be released by a quick tug. Some needles are eyed allowing the surgeon to choose the needle and suture material to suit the job, but these are less common. In gynaecology, eyed Mayo needles tend only to be used by some surgeons to suspend the vault following vaginal hysterectomy.

The Body

The body is the section of the needle grasped by the needle holder. The diameter should be as close as possible to that of the suture material being used in order to minimise trauma. Whilst straight needles are useful for skin, curved needles are more common (Figure 6.2). The curvature varies depending on the tissue being sutured and is expressed as eighths of a circle. The commonest are

How to Perform Operative Procedures in Obstetrics and Gynaecology, First Edition.
Edited by Wai Yoong, Abha Govind, and Wasim Lodhi.
© 2020 John Wiley & Sons Ltd. Published 2020 by John Wiley & Sons Ltd.
Companion website: www.wiley.com/go/yoong/obgyn

½ curve (half circle) and 3/8. In general, the deeper the plane the more curved the needle should be. J needles are 'J shaped' and can be used to close deeper tissues such as the rectus sheath after laparoscopy.

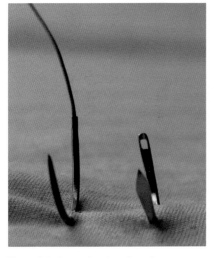

Figure 6.1 Swaged and eyed needles.

The Point

The point extends from the extreme point of the needle to the maximum diameter of the body and different points are designed to give the required amount of cutting for different tissues. The commonest needles used in gynaecological surgery include the following (Figure 6.3).

- **Blunt points** are used for blunt dissection and suturing friable tissue. Blunt points are also used in patients with blood-borne viruses as they reduce the chance of needle stick injuries. The symbol used to represent this needle is a small circle inside a larger one.
- **Tapered points** are used for soft, easily penetrable tissue. The symbol used is a circle with a dot inside.
- **Taper-cuttings** are used to cut through most tissues with minimal trauma. The symbol used is a circle with a dot inside and three converging lines.
- **Cuttings** are used for cutting tougher, more difficult-to-penetrate tissues. The symbol used is a triangle.

(a)

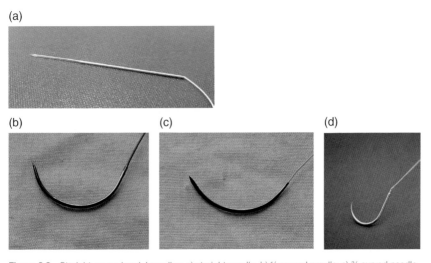

(b)   (c)   (d)

Figure 6.2 Straight, curved and J needles: a) straight needle, b) ½ curved needle, c) ¾ curved needle, d) J needle.

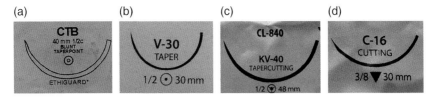

(a)   (b)   (c)   (d)

Figure 6.3 Different needle points: a) blunt, b) tapered point, c) taper-cutting, d) cutting.

Sutures

The time taken to heal and regain tensile strength varies between different tissues. It is this principle that guides the choice of suture for any given procedure – the suture must retain its tensile strength until the point the tissue has healed sufficiently to remain opposed unsupported. It may then be beneficial for the suture to be reabsorbed to prevent a long-term foreign body. Sutures vary in size, strength and material.

Suture Sizes

Suture sizing is a little confusing for historical reasons. The system originally sized sutures from 1 to 6, with 1 being the thinnest and 6 being the thickest. As thinner sutures were developed, they were named 0, then 2–0, 3–0, etc. Modern sutures range from number 5 (0.7 mm) used in orthopaedics to 11–0 (0.01 mm) used in ophthalmic surgery (Figure 6.4). Thicker number 1 sutures are commonly used to close the uterus at Caesarean section, whereas thinner 2–0 sutures are used when repairing the perineum.

Choice of Suture

Different tissues take different amounts of time to heal and this may be prolonged by any comorbidities or infections present (Figure 6.5). It is important to remember that tissue will never regain its original

Suture size	Diameter in mm
11-0	0.01
10-0	0.02
9-0	0.03
8-0	0.04
7-0	0.05
6-0	0.07
5-0	0.1
4-0	0.15
3-0	0.2
2-0	0.3
0	0.35
1	0.4
2	0.5
3	0.6
4	0.6
5	0.7

Figure 6.4 Suture sizes.

Tissue	Healing Time
Skin	1–2 weeks
Subcutaneous tissue	2 weeks
Peritoneum	4–10 days
Uterus	8 days
Vagina and perineum	8–10 days
Bladder	5 days
Ligaments tendons	6 weeks

Figure 6.5 Healing times of different tissues.

tensile strength after healing. This is particularly relevant in obstetrics where women often present in labour having had a previous Caesarean section.

(a)   (b)

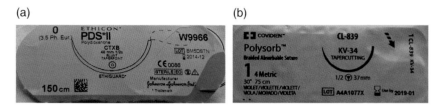

Figure 6.6 Commonly used absorbable sutures: a) monofilament, e.g. PDS, b) multifilament, e.g. Vicryl.

(a)   (b)

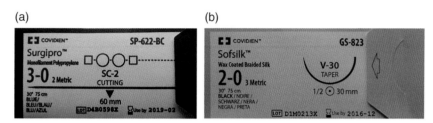

Figure 6.7 Commonly used non-absorbable sutures: a) monofilament, e.g. Prolene, b) multifilament, e.g. silk.

Sutures can be broadly divided into absorbable and non-absorbable and then further subdivided into monofilament and multifilament. Monofilament is made from a single strand giving it the advantages of tying down smoothly and with less risk of harbouring microorganisms. Multifilament suture is made from several strands twisted or braided together giving it good handling and tying properties.

The most commonly used absorbable sutures in obstetrics and gynaecology are PDS and Vicryl (Figure 6.6). PDS is commonly used to repair the anal sphincter after a 3rd degree tear as it is monofilament suture which helps prevent infection. Vicryl is a multifilament suture and therefore easier to handle and tie. It is used frequently for closing the uterus and rectus sheath at Caesarean section. Vicryl rapide has the same properties but is absorbed more quickly and is therefore useful in tissues that heal quickly and when a long-term foreign body is not desired. Vicryl rapide is used to repair first- and second-degree perineal tears and in vaginal surgery.

The most commonly used non-absorbable sutures are Prolene and silk (Figure 6.7). Prolene is a monofilament suture which is commonly used for skin closure after laparotomy. Silk is a multifilament suture often used to secure surgical drains.

Specialised Sutures

The Endoloop ligature facilitates the ligation of pedicles in laparoscopic procedures. It consists of an 18″ long ligature in a plastic tube that is narrow at one end and scored at the other, where it is attached. Once the ligature is in place, the scored end is simply snapped and pulled upward to tighten the loop and secure the knot. Multifilament/braided sutures such as Mersilene tape have been traditionally used for cervical cerclage and will be covered in that chapter.

PART II

Obstetrics

7 Assisted Vaginal Delivery

Natasha Barbaneagra, Katie Andersen, and Wasim Lodhi

Video Duration | 7 mins 41 secs

Overview

Skill in forceps and ventouse delivery remains an integral part of modern obstetric practice as at least 10% of deliveries are assisted using these instruments. The authors discuss indications, prerequisites and technical tips on how to conduct assisted vaginal deliveries safely.

Introduction

Instrumental vaginal deliveries can potentially harm both mother and baby and so should be undertaken with care. However, a second-stage Caesarean section is not a substitute for instrumental vaginal deliveries as it can be extremely difficult to perform and is associated with high morbidity and implications for future births.

Various techniques may help **reduce instrumental delivery rates,** such as one-to-one support in labour, upright/lateral positions in labour, use of a partogram, avoidance of epidural analgesia, delayed pushing and active management of the second stage of labour with oxytocin for nulliparous women with epidurals.

Classification of Assisted Vaginal Delivery

OUTLET

Fetal scalp visible without separating the labia.

Fetal skull has reached the pelvic floor.

Fetal head is at or on the perineum.

Sagittal suture is in the anterior–posterior diameter or right or left occiput.

LOW

Leading point of the skull (not caput) is at station plus 2 or more and not on the pelvic floor.

MID

Fetal head is no more than 1/5th palpable per abdomen.

How to Perform Operative Procedures in Obstetrics and Gynaecology, First Edition.
Edited by Wai Yoong, Abha Govind, and Wasim Lodhi.
© 2020 John Wiley & Sons Ltd. Published 2020 by John Wiley & Sons Ltd.
Companion website: www.wiley.com/go/yoong/obgyn

Leading point of the skull is above the level of ischial spines plus 2 but not above the spines.

HIGH

Operative vaginal delivery is not recommended where the head is 2/5th or more palpable abdominally and the presenting part is above the level of the ischial spines.

Indications for Assisted Vaginal Delivery

FETAL

Presumed fetal compromise.

MATERNAL

To shorten and reduce the effects of the second stage of labour in medical conditions (cardiac disease class III or IV, hypertensive crises, myasthenia gravis, spinal cord injury patients, proliferative retinopathy).

INADEQUATE PROGRESS IN THE SECOND STAGE OF LABOUR

Nulliparous women – lack of continuing progress for three hours with regional anaesthesia, or two hours without regional anaesthesia.

Multiparous women – lack of continuing progress for two hours with regional anaesthesia, or one hour without regional anaesthesia.

Maternal fatigue/exhaustion.

Choice of Instruments for Assisted Vaginal Delivery

Conditions Where Ventouse Delivery Would Be Preferred over Forceps

1 Urgent low lift-out delivery with no previous analgesia.

2 Rotational delivery.

3 Operator or maternal preference, when either instrument would be suitable.

Conditions Where Forceps Would Be Preferred to Ventouse Delivery

1 Poor maternal effort.

2 Operator or maternal preference, when either instrument would be suitable.

3 Large amount of caput.

4 Gestation of less than 34 weeks (at 34–36 weeks of gestation, ventouse is relatively contraindicated).

5 Marked active bleeding from a fetal blood-sampling site.

6 After-coming head of the breech.

7 Face presentation.

Prerequisites for Assisted Vaginal Delivery

Full abdominal and vaginal examination

- Head is 1/5th or less palpable per abdomen.
- Vertex presentation.
- Cervix is fully dilated and the membranes ruptured.
- Exact position of the head should be determined so that safe and correct placement of the instrument can be achieved.
- Assessment of caput and moulding.
- Adequate pelvis,

Preparation of mother

- Clear explanation and informed consent obtained.
- Appropriate analgesia for mid-cavity rotational deliveries: regional block or a pudendal block,
- Maternal bladder is emptied.
- Aseptic technique.

Preparation of staff

- Operator must have the knowledge, experience and necessary skill.
- Adequate facilities available.
- Back-up plan in place in case of failure to deliver. A senior obstetrician competent in performing mid-cavity deliveries should be present if a junior trainee is performing the delivery.

- Anticipation of complications that may arise – shoulder dystocia, postpartum haemorrhage, failed instrumental delivery ('when to stop').
- Personnel present that are trained in neonatal resuscitation.

Conducting Forceps Delivery

Operator **assembles the instrument** to ensure that both the blades lock and are part of a pair.

Patient is placed in dorsal **lithotomy** position. Abdominal examination is performed to ensure that no more than 1/5th of the fetal head is palpable per abdomen (Figure 7.1). Confirm the position of the presenting part by palpating for the fontanelles (Figure 7.2). Appropriate **analgesia** (either pudendal block/regional anaesthesia) is administered (Figure 7.3). Two types of forceps delivery are commonly practised in the United Kingdom: these are mid-cavity using **Neville Barnes** forceps (or similar instrument) and outlet forceps using **Wrigley** forceps. Some operators still perform Kielland's rotational forceps but this is beyond the scope of this chapter.

It is important to **explain** the indication and procedure to woman and take a verbal/written consent for instrumental delivery as well as for the possibility of an episiotomy.

The operator introduces the right hand in to the vagina with the palm of the hand facing medially towards the fetal head. Traditionally, **the left blade** of the forceps is introduced first. The handle of left blade should be almost parallel to the right inguinal region of the mother and the blade gently inserted by sliding it over the right palm of operator's hand after applying lubrication (Figure 7.4). The tips of the operator's fingers guard and guide the forceps blade during insertion, which should be done with minimal force.

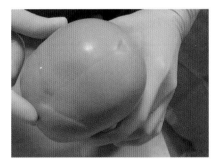

Figure 7.2   Confirm position of the fetal head.

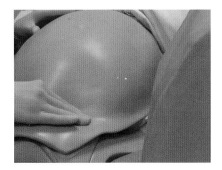

Figure 7.1   Per abdominal examination to ensure that no more than 1/5th of fetal head is palpable.

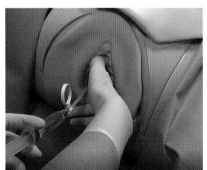

Figure 7.3   Pudendal nerve infiltration for analgesia.

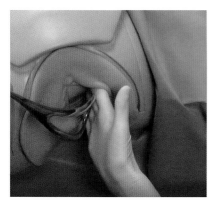

Figure 7.4 The left Neville Barnes forceps blade is introduced first by sliding along the inner aspect of the operator's right palm.

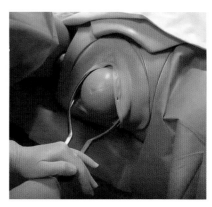

Figure 7.6 Pajot's manoeuvre to guide the fetal head through the Curve of Carus.

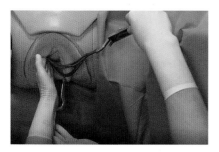

Figure 7.5 A similar manoeuvre is repeated with the contralateral forceps blade.

Following application of the left blade, the operator checks that it sits comfortably in the hollow of the pelvis. The operator's **left** hand is then placed in the vagina and **the right blade** slipped medial to this in a similar manner as the contralateral side (Figure 7.5).

Once both blades are in position, they are gently locked. If the blades do not lock, the application is rechecked: **never** try to **force the blades** into position!

Gentle traction is applied **whilst** the mother is **pushing** with uterine contractions.

Pajot's manoeuvre is often used with the non-dominant hand applying downward pressure to follow the Curve of Carus whilst the dominant hand maintains traction (Figure 7.6). **Episiotomy** is performed if there is substantial risk of tearing when the fetal head distends the perineum.

Once the head is delivered, the right blade is disengaged and removed, followed by the left. The delivery of the body is completed in a normal manner, allowing for restitution and rotation of the trunk.

Conducting Ventouse Delivery

The most commonly used vacuum cup is the Kiwi Omnicup (Clinical Innovations).

After vaginal examination, the cup is applied with the ridge facing towards fetal occiput. This acts as a marker to confirm fetal head rotation. It is important to identify the **flexion point** which is **3 cm** anterior to posterior fontanelle. The centre of the Kiwi cup should be placed over the flexion point (Figure 7.7). Kiwi cup tubing has prominent **black markers** at **6 and 11 cm** position: the purpose of these is to assist the operator in the correct placement of the

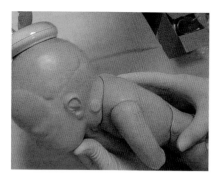

Figure 7.7 Kiwi Omnicup being applied to the flexion point 3 cm anterior to the posterior fontanelle.

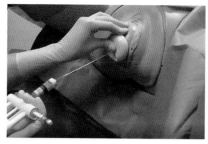

Figure 7.8 The operator's dominant hand applying traction whilst the other hand provides support to the cup and assesses the descent of the fetal head.

Kiwi Omnicup. In cases of **occipito-posterior position,** the distance between the flexion point and introitus is likely to be 11 cm, whilst in occipito-anterior position, this is likely to be 6 cm. This is approximated using the fingers during digital examination.

The cup is lubricated using **KY jelly** or obstetric cream and is inserted through the introitus by stretching the perineum posteriorly to create space. Once the cup is placed over the flexion point, vacuum is generated to **150 mmHg** by pumping the handle of the device. The edges of the cup are palpated to confirm that no **maternal tissue** is inadvertently trapped. Once the operator is satisfied with the correct placement, the vacuum is increased to **400–600 mmHg**.

Gentle traction is applied as soon as a contraction starts and in conjunction with maternal effort. Traction supports maternal pushing and the expulsive efforts of uterine contractions. If uterine contractions are infrequent or weak, **augmentation with oxytocin** infusion should be considered. The direction of traction is initially **downwards** and then along the **axis of the pelvis** (Curve of Carus) as the fetal head

starts to descend. The operator's dominant hand applies traction whilst the other hand provides **support** to the **cup** and assesses the descent of the fetal head (Figure 7.8). Episiotomy may be indicated if the perineum does not stretch adequately when the head distends the introitus. Once the head is delivered, the vacuum is released and cup removed.

After Delivery

- If the baby is delivered in good condition, then he or she should be handed over to the mother as soon as possible to encourage skin-to-skin contact.
- Double-clamp the cord and take paired **cord blood** samples.
- Deliver the placenta by controlled cord traction when signs of placental separation occur.
- **Check for perineal damage** with particular attention for the integrity of anal sphincter and anal mucosa.
- Repair the perineal tear or episiotomy.
- Once the repairs are completed, a vaginal and rectal examination should be performed to confirm restoration of anatomy.
- Check **swab, needle** and **instrument counts.**

- Examine the baby's head to confirm that the position of the instrument used was correct for self-audit.
- **Document** clearly.
- Prescribe analgesia/thromboprophylaxis as needed.
- Provide advice on bladder care.
- **Debrief** the woman and the team.

Further Reading

American College of Obstetricians and Gynecologists (2000). *ACOG Practice Bulletin No 17: Operative Vaginal Delivery*. Washington DC: USA.

RCOG (2011). Operative Vaginal Delivery (Green-top Guideline No. 26). Published: 01/02/2011 www.rcog.org.uk/globalassets/documents/guidelines/gtg_26.pdf.

8 Caesarean Section

Sayantana Das and Abha Govind

Video Duration | 9 mins 22 secs

Overview

Caesarean section (CS) is one of the **most common** operative interventions in obstetrics and the majority of trainees will be familiar with this procedure. The authors discuss the indications and present a standardised way of doing CS.

Introduction

The inappropriate use of CS can have major implications for maternal morbidity and mortality. It is therefore important to discuss the risks and benefits of CS and vaginal birth with women, taking into account their circumstances, concerns, priorities and plans for future pregnancies (including the risks of placental problems with multiple CS) (NICE 2019).

Indications

The most common indications include **previous CS, fetal hypoxia, dystocia** in labour, **breech** presentation at term, **maternal medical** conditions (such as cardiac disease), diabetes, severe pre-eclampsia and finally **low-lying placenta.**

Degree of Urgency

The urgency of CS should be documented using the following standardised scheme in order to aid clear communication between healthcare professionals about the urgency of a CS:

Category 1: Immediate threat to the life of the women or fetus. To be done within 30 minutes.

Category 2: Maternal/fetal compromise which is not immediately life threatening. To be done within 60 minutes.

Category 3: No maternal/fetal compromise but early delivery needed. To be done within 75 minutes.

Category 4: Procedure planned to suit mother and staff.

Procedure

A regional anaesthetic block is inserted. The patient is placed in the **dorsal** position and a **Foley** catheter is inserted. The abdomen is then cleaned and draped. The pubic symphysis is palpated and a **transverse incision** is made just below the pubic hair line, approximately 2 cm above the pubic symphysis. The abdomen

How to Perform Operative Procedures in Obstetrics and Gynaecology, First Edition.
Edited by Wai Yoong, Abha Govind, and Wasim Lodhi.
© 2020 John Wiley & Sons Ltd. Published 2020 by John Wiley & Sons Ltd.
Companion website: www.wiley.com/go/yoong/obgyn

is opened through a lower transverse incision (Pfannensteil or modified Cohen) (Figure 8.1). After opening the peritoneal cavity, the uterus is checked for dexo or levo rotation. The bladder is retracted with a **Doyen's** retractor. The **vesico-uterine fold** of the peritoneum is identified (Figure 8.2). This is the part of the peritoneum attached to the surface of the uterus and is the upper margin of the lower uterine segment. The peritoneum is divided 2–3 cm below the level of this attachment in the midline and extend laterally on each side. A scalpel is used and with gentle horizontal stokes a **2 cm incision** made on the uterus. A forefinger or scalpel handle is used to burrow through the final thin layer. Once the uterus is entered, the forefinger is placed between the fetus and uterine muscle towards one side and curved Mayo scissors are used for sharp dissection for 2 cm on each side. The incision is extended laterally using **the surgeon's fingers**: try to do this symmetrically so as to avoid extension on one side. The fetal **head** is grasped placing the flat of the hand downwards between the head and lower uterine segment. **Wrigley's forceps** can be used when the fetal head is high; the left blade is inserted below the baby's head and the right blade anteriorly. The blades should **lock** and the head be delivered via the uterine incision. After removing the Doyens retractor, the assistant applies **fundal pressure** to aid **delivery of** the baby. The placenta is delivered by controlled cord traction. The incised edges are held with **Green-Armytage** tissue forceps and the angles are secured bilaterally (Figure 8.3). A **continuous suture** with Vicryl 1 in a running fashion is used to repair the myometrium (Figure 8.4). The repair is conventionally done in two layers and the second layer, which can also be continuous, is used to bury and support the inner

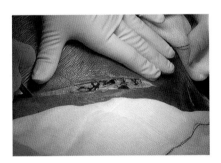

Figure 8.1 Opening the abdomen through a lower transverse incision.

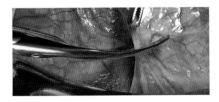

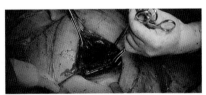

Figure 8.3 The incised myometrial edges are held using Green-Armytage tissue forceps.

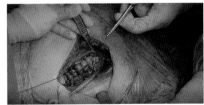

Figure 8.2 Identifying the vesico-uterine fold of peritoneum.

Figure 8.4 Repairing the uterus in two layers.

layer of repair. Take care not to go beyond the already tied uterine angle. Additional haemostatic sutures may be required if there are bleeding points.

The **ovaries** and fallopian tubes are inspected for any abnormalities after cleaning the **paracolic gutters.** The **rectus** sheath is reconstructed with continuous suture. Subcutaneous fat can be closed with interrupted or continuous suture if more than 2 cm thick. The skin is usually approximated using a subcuticular suture. The vagina is cleaned using a 'swab on a stick' and any bleeding noted. **The surgical team** then signs out using the WHO Checklist.

Delivery of a Baby Presenting as Breech during CS

Following the uterine incision, **grasp** the fetal **legs** with one hand and assist the delivery of the extended legs with flexion. Ensure that the **fetal back** remains anterior in order to prevent hyperextension of the fetal head later. Grasp the thighs with the **thumb** over the **sacrum** and inner finger around the iliac crest. Gently apply traction to deliver the body until the **nape of the neck** is visible. The baby's body is then rotated 180° each side to deliver both arms – this is called **Lovset's manoeuvre.** The delivery of the head then follows the delivery of the trunk. The **Mauriceau Smellie Veit** manoeuvre may be used to deliver an extended fetal head. The head is delivered by placing the forefinger and middle finger on either side of the maxilla to promote **flexion** of the fetal **head.** The body of the baby is placed on the operator's hand with a leg on each side.

Further Reading

NHS Choices (2019). Overview: Caesarean Section. www.nhs.uk/Conditions/Caesarean-section/Pages/Introduction.aspx

NICE (2019). National Institute for Health and Care Excellence: Clinical guideline [CG132]. Published date: November 2011 updated: September 2019 www.nice.org.uk/guidance/cg132/informationforpublic.

RCOG (2015). Choosing to have a Caesarean Section. https://www.rcog.org.uk/en/patients/patient-leaflets/choosing-to-have-a-caesarean-section/.

9 Uterine Compression Sutures for Uterine Atony

Wai Yoong and Wasim Lodhi

Video Duration | 7 mins 3 secs

Overview

The ability to insert compression sutures in the surgical management of atonic postpartum haemorrhage (PPH) is important to the obstetrician. The vertical compression sutures described in this chapter are the best known and easiest to perform.

Introduction

PPH remains the commonest cause of maternal death worldwide and was responsible for 12 **maternal deaths** in the last Confidential Enquiry into Maternal and Child Health (Norman 2011). Previously, surgical management of PPH included intrauterine **balloon tamponade, uterine and internal iliac vessel ligation,** culminating in **subtotal abdominal hysterectomy.** The current generation of new consultant obstetricians needs to be familiar and confident with the application of **uterine compression sutures** as a **conservative** surgical intervention for **atonic** PPH. We will be describing and demonstrating how to perform two of the most commonly used compression sutures as well as a combination technique of compression sutures and uterine balloon tamponade ('the uterine sandwich').

B-Lynch Suture

Suture material suggested: Monocryl no 1 on a 90 mm blunt needle (Ethicon).

The concept of vertical **brace** suture to generate **compressive pressure** on an atonic uterus was first described by Professor B-Lynch and colleagues in their seminal *British Journal of Obstetrics and Gynaecology* paper in 1997. A **laparotomy** is necessary to exteriorise the uterus. A **lower uterine segment** incision is made in the uterus unless an existing incision is already present from a Caesarean section (CS) delivery: this is to ensure that the cavity is totally devoid of placental segments or clots.

How to Perform Operative Procedures in Obstetrics and Gynaecology, First Edition.
Edited by Wai Yoong, Abha Govind, and Wasim Lodhi.
© 2020 John Wiley & Sons, Ltd. Published 2020 by John Wiley & Sons, Ltd.
Companion website: www.wiley.com/go/yoong/obgyn

Test for Potential Success of B-Lynch Suture before Performing the Procedure

After placing the patient in **Lloyd Davies** (frog leg) **position,** with an assistant between her legs to intermittently **swab the vagina,** the uterus is **exteriorised** and **bimanual compression** performed by the surgeon. The uterus is compressed by placing **one hand posteriorly** with the ends of the accoucher's **fingers at the level** of **cervix** and the other hand bunched up as a **fist below** the **bladder reflection.**

Procedure

Professor B-Lynch, the originator of this suture, is very precise about entry and exit points. With the bladder displaced inferiorly, **Monocryl no 1 suture is** inserted **3 cm below the CS incision** on the patient's left side and threaded **through the** uterine **cavity** to emerge **3 cm above the upper incision** margin, approximately **4 cm from the lateral border** of the uterus. Once situated over the fundus, the suture should be **vertical** and lie about **4 cm from the cornu.** The entry point for suture on the **posterior** surface of the uterus is at the **insertion of** the **uterosacral ligament approximately** at the **level of** the **uterine incision.** The suture enters **within** the **cavity** side of the posterior uterine wall. The suture is then guided laterally and exits the cavity at the level of the right uterosacral ligament and goes over the **top of the fundus** and onto the anterior surface of the uterus on the right side. The **needle re-enters** the cavity at a point 3 cm above the upper uterine incision and 4 cm from the lateral side of the uterus. It finally exits 3 cm below the lower uterine incision margin on the right side after which tension is applied to compress the uterus (Figure 9.1).

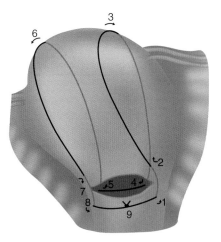

Figure 9.1 The B-Lynch Suture comprising nine steps.

The assistant **maintains compressive pressure** as the suture material is tightened through from its different portals to ensure **uniform tension** and no slippage. The two ends of the suture are pulled securely and a **double throw knot** is placed for security to **maintain tension** after the lower segment incision has been closed by either the one- or two-layer method. We always **hold the first knot** (as shown in the video footage) with **Spencer-Wells forceps** so that tension in the suture is maintained before the second throw is made and tightened.

The assistant standing between the patient's legs **swabs** the **vagina** again and can **confirm** that the **bleeding** has been **controlled**.

Hayman Suture

First described by Hayman et al. (2002), this technique is **simpler** to perform, with **fewer steps** to remember than the B-Lynch suture.

Suggested suture material: Monocryl 1 on a 90 mm blunt needle (Ethicon).

Procedure

This technique does not require making an incision in the uterus. Whilst there are no randomised control trials against the B-Lynch suture, anecdotal evidence (Hayman et al. 2002; Ghezzi et al. 2007) suggest that the two techniques have similar efficacy.

The bladder is reflected downward and Monocryl No 1 90mm blunt needle is inserted through the **anterior wall** of the lower uterine segment below the CS incision and approximately 1 cm above the bladder reflection. The blunt needle exits through the posterior wall near the uterosacral ligament. From the exit point in the posterior wall, the suture is then brought to the fundus and a surgical knot secured at the top of the fundus. A second No.1 Monocryl needle is used in the same manner as the first on the contralateral side. The two vertical sutures are thus parallel to each other. After placing the sutures, the knots are tied as tightly as possible to compress the lower segment of the uterine cavity by apposing the anterior and posterior walls, again using Spencer-Wells forceps to hold the first knot in order to maintain tension, before the second knot is thrown and tightened (Figure 9.2).

The Combination Technique of Compression Suture and Uterine Balloon Tamponade ('The Uterine Sandwich')

Suture material suggested: Monocryl no 1 blunt needle (Ethicon).

The combination of vertical **compression sutures** and intrauterine **balloon tamponade** was first described by Danso and Reginald (2002) and two subsequent case series (Nelson and O'Brien 2007; Yoong et al. 2012) have also been published in the literature.

Procedure

The B-Lynch and Hayman sutures were applied as described by the original authors (B-Lynch et al. 1997; Hayman et al. 2002) with the uterus exteriorised but using the absorbable Monocryl 1/0 suture on a 90mm curved ethigard blunt needle (Ethicon) instead of No 2. chromic catgut or 2 Dexon (Covidien, Gosport, UK).

Where a uterine incision was already present, the **Bakri balloon** was **introduced abdominally via the incision** and the **caudal end** then **pulled through the cervix** into the vagina by an assistant. Only when the compression sutures as primary surgical procedures failed to control bleeding were the balloons then inflated to the appropriate volumes.

The compression sutures are placed prior to the introduction of the balloons in order to reduce the risk of puncturing the latter. To facilitate suture placement, the atonic uterus is bimanually compressed by the assistant to reduce its thickness and we recommend **straightening the curve of the needle** to ensure that it is able to

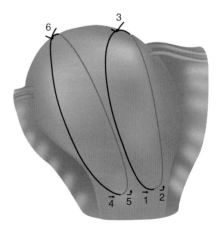

Figure 9.2 The Hayman suture comprising six steps: two separate parallel vertical sutures are placed to apply compression to the uterus.

penetrate the combined thickness of the anterior and posterior walls of the lower segment. The Bakri balloon was inflated to a volume not exceeding 350 ml (median 300 ml) to exert **counterpressure** after the appropriate tension was applied by pulling taut the two lengths of the compression sutures (Figure 9.3). Insufflation of the balloon was **stopped** when there was subjective visual evidence of **undue blanching** of the uterus. The risk of the balloon migrating through the cervix was reduced by **packing the vaginal canal** with iodine-soaked gauze, which also has the effect of increasing tamponade on the lower segment.

Tips

- Have a schematic diagram of compression sutures laminated and available for reference in the labour ward theatre.
- Use the 'double needle holder' technique as shown in the DVD footage: this makes the needle more stable, thus easier to go through the thick uterine walls (Figure 9.4).
- Use Monocryl no 1 suture on a large 90 mm curved needle.
- Bimanually compress the uterus while tightening the suture.

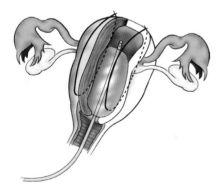

Figure 9.3 'Uterine sandwich' technique combining external vertical compression suture with intrauterine Bakri balloon tamponade. *Source*: Reproduced with permission of Dhanuson Dharmasena.

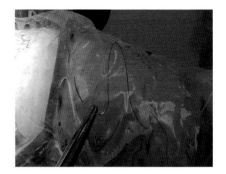

Figure 9.4 Using two needle holders to grasp the needle securely.

- Use Spencer-Wells forceps to hold the first knot of the compression suture to maintain tension.
- Beware of the small risk of uterine necrosis: use vertical compression sutures only, not vertical plus horizontal (Figure 9.4)

Complications

Uterine necrosis is the rare complication of these techniques.

Further Reading

B-Lynch, C., Coker, A., Lawal, A.H. et al. (1997). The B-Lynch surgical technique for the control of massive postpartum haemorrhage: an alternative to hysterectomy? Five cases reported. *BJOG* 104: 372–375.

Danso, D. and Reginald, P. (2002). Combined B-Lynch suture with intrauterine balloon catheter triumphs over massive postpartum haemorrhage. *BJOG* 109 (8): 963.

Ghezzi, F., Cromi, A., Raio, L. et al. (2007). The Hayman technique: a simple method to treat postpartum haemorrhage. *BJOG* 114: 362–365.

Hayman, R.G., Arulkumaran, S., and Steer, P. (2002). Uterine compressions sutures: surgical management of postpartum haemorrhage. *Obstet. Gynecol.* 99: 502–506.

Nelson, W.L. and O'Brien, J.M. (2007). The uterine sandwich for persistent uterine atony: combining the B-Lynch compression suture and an intrauterine Bakri balloon. *Am. J. Obstet. Gynecol.* 196 (5): e9–e10.

Norman, J. (2011). Haemorrhage. In: saving Mothers' lives CEMACE 2006-8. (Lewis G, ed). Chapter 4. *BJOG* 118 (suppl 1): 1–203.

Yoong, W., Ridout, A., Memtsa, M. et al. (2012). Application of uterine compression suture in association with intrauterine balloon tamponade ("uterine sandwich") for postpartum hemorrhage: case series of 11 patients. *Acta Obstet. Gynecol. Scand.* 91 (1): 147–151.

10 Cervical Cerclage

Joan Bager, Dhanuson Dharmasena, and Wai Yoong

Video Duration | 5 mins 52 secs

Overview

Knowledge of when to offer cervical cerclage (McDonald and Shirodkar techniques) and how to perform the techniques are described in this chapter.

Introduction

Cervical cerclage is usually performed as a **prophylactic** measure in asymptomatic women and inserted **electively** at **12–14** weeks of gestation. Traditionally this was inserted as a treatment for **mid-trimester loss** (from 16^{+0} weeks of pregnancy onwards) attributed to **cervical incompetence** but common contemporary indications include **spontaneous preterm birth** (up to 34^{+0} weeks of pregnancy) due to **multiple pregnancy, uterine anomalies**, a history of cervical trauma (e.g. **conisation** or operations requiring **forced dilatation** of the cervical canal) and **cervical shortening** (between 16^{+0} and 24^{+0} weeks of pregnancy that show a cervical length of 25 mm or less) seen on sonographic examination.

It is debatable whether cervical cerclage should be recommended in women without a history of spontaneous preterm delivery or second-trimester loss who have an incidentally identified **short cervix of 25 mm or less** on ultrasonography.

Rescue or emergency cerclage refers to the insertion of cerclage as a salvage measure in the case of premature cervical dilatation with or without **exposed fetal membranes** in the vagina. This may be discovered by ultrasound examination of the cervix or as a result of a **speculum/ physical examination** performed for symptoms such as vaginal discharge, bleeding or 'sensation of pressure'. **Advanced dilatation** of the cervix (**more than 4 cm**) or membrane prolapse beyond the external os appears to be associated with a high chance of **cerclage failure.** In the absence of clinical signs of **chorioamnionitis**, rescue cerclage **must not be delayed** and **inflammatory markers** such as maternal white cell count and C-reactive protein can be done to help decide the appropriateness of rescue cerclage.

How to Perform Operative Procedures in Obstetrics and Gynaecology, First Edition.
Edited by Wai Yoong, Abha Govind, and Wasim Lodhi.
© 2020 John Wiley & Sons Ltd. Published 2020 by John Wiley & Sons Ltd.
Companion website: www.wiley.com/go/yoong/obgyn

The authors will demonstrate the **McDonald and Shirodkar cervical sutures** as these are the most commonly practised procedures. Transabdominal and laparoscopic approaches which involve placing the suture at the cervico-isthmic junction are beyond the scope of this chapter.

Operative Procedure

Elective transvaginal cerclage can safely be performed as a **day-case** procedure and there is **no evidence** to support the use of routine perioperative **tocolysis** in women undergoing insertion of cerclage. The decision for **antibiotic prophylaxis** at the time of cerclage placement should be at the discretion of the operating team.

The procedure is performed in the **lithotomy position** under **general or spinal** anaesthesia. Access is crucial and this is made easier if the surgeon and assistants are sitting down as shown (Figure 10.1). After routine preparation, draping and bladder catheterisation, retraction labial sutures are placed and an Auvard vaginal speculum sutured in to enable access to the vagina and cervix. A **double needled Mersilene tape** (Ethicon RS22) is normally utilised (Figure 10.2) and the authors routinely use **two needle holders** (Figure 10.3) to grasp the needle as shown in the video footage to maximise stability when inserting the suture.

McDonald Suture

For the McDonald technique, a **purse-string suture** is placed at the **cervicovaginal junction**, without bladder mobilisation, **starting** at the **12 o'clock** position (Figure 10.4). The cervix is held with atraumatic **sponge forceps** at 12 and

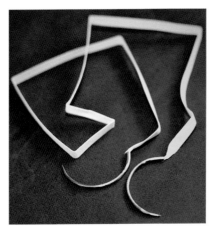

Figure 10.2 Mersilene tape.

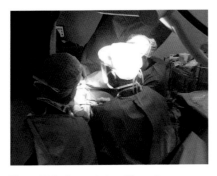

Figure 10.1 Suggested positions of surgeons when performing cervical cerclage.

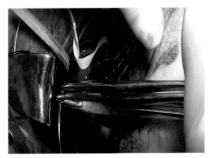

Figure 10.3 The needle is held securely with two needle holders.

6 o'clock for stabilisation and gentle traction. The needle is then pushed through to **exit at 9 o'clock** position, using wrist supination and following the natural curve of the needle to facilitate entry and exit of the tip of the needle. The **proximal needle holder** is then removed and used to grasp and pull through the needle, whilst the second needle holder is released. The **second bite** is taken at 9 o'clock to exit at the **6 o'clock** position, making sure that there is minimal gap between the 9 o'clock exit and re-insertion points. This is repeated at 6 o'clock and **3 o'clock** positions, so that the final exit point is close to the initial entry at 12 o'clock position. Both needles are then cut and the tape is tightened to ensure that the internal cervical os is no longer incompetent: the surgeon can verify this by placing the index finger in the os. A double surgeon's **knot** is then thrown at the **12 o'clock** position, using the index finger

to push down the knot to ensure that it is secure. A second and third knot is then placed on top of the first and a 1–2 cm **loop** is often made to facilitate removal of the tape. This is depicted as Figure 10.5 in the coronal section.

Shirodkar Suture

A high transvaginal cerclage (**Shirodkar**) may be indicated **if the McDonald** technique used in a previous pregnancy has been **unsuccessful**. A Shirodkar purse-string suture is placed following **bladder mobilisation** to allow insertion above the level of the cardinal ligaments, above the internal cervical os. The authors describe a **modified version,** which involves less dissection.

The cervix is held with a sponge holding forceps on the anterior and posterior cervical lips. A solution of 20 ml of bupivacaine 0.5% w/v and adrenaline 1 : 200 000 is

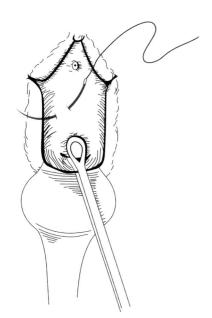

Figure 10.4 Mersilene tape with 5 mm needle inserted at 12 o'clock.

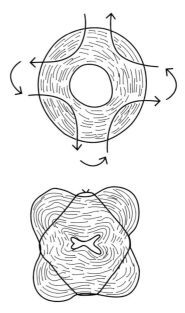

Figure 10.5 Coronal plane showing McDonald suture when tightened.

injected into the anterior and posterior fornices to help separate tissue planes and to promote vasoconstriction. A **3 cm transverse incision** with the blade is made in the **anterior vaginal wall** where the vaginal skin meets the cervix (from 9 o'clock to 3 o'clock) to expose the cervix (Figure 10.6). The cervix is separated from the bladder using **blunt dissection** with a swab against the surgeon's index finger. A similar **incision** is repeated on the **posterior fornix,** from 8 o'clock to 4 o'clock, exposing the cervix on the posterior aspect. The surgeon's finger and thumb then **pinch and compress** the paracervical tissue anteroposteriorly just lateral to the cervix. A needle attached to Mersilene tape is then directed between the lateral aspect of the cervix and the **compressed paracervical tissues** from the lateral border of the anterior forniceal incision and the posterior forniceal incision (Figure 10.7). The procedure is then repeated in the **reverse direction** and the same needle is passed postero-anteriorly from the lateral aspect of the posterior incision to the anterior incision.

The **double needle holder** technique helps stabilise the needle as it traverses the paracervical tissues. The two ends of the tape are then crossed in front of the cervix and the **knot** placed flush with the

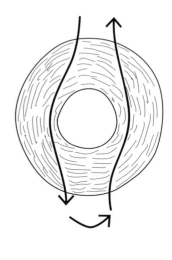

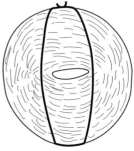

Figure 10.7 Coronal plane depicting Shirodkar suture when tightened.

cervix at the **level of the internal os**. The ends of the knot are then cut. Continuous **2/0 Vicryl** is used to close the posterior incision completely. The anterior incision is closed in two separate halves, with the end of the Mersilene tape protruding in the midline: this can later be cut when the pregnancy reaches 37 completed weeks.

Rescue Cerclage

For **rescue cerclage,** the patient is placed in a **steep head-down** position to help reduce bulging membranes. **Two sponge forceps** are placed on the anterior lip of the cervix and a further two on the posterior

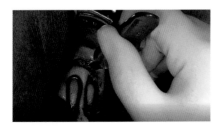

Figure 10.6 Shirodkar suture showing transverse incision on the anterior vaginal wall.

lip; gentle traction is then applied to see if the cervix can be carefully pulled over to cover the membranes. **A 22-gauge Foley catheter** is inserted through the cervix and slowly inflated with **20–30 ml of saline** which further acts to reduce the membranes; the surgeon's **index finger** is placed in the cervix to ensure that membranes are safely away from the field of surgery. Either the **McDonald or Shirodkar technique** can be used to insert the cerclage as described above.

Post-Operative Management

Bed rest in women who have undergone cerclage should not be routinely recommended, but the decision can be individualised, taking into account the clinical circumstances and the potential adverse effects that bed rest could have on women and their families, in addition to increased costs for the healthcare system.

Abstinence from sexual intercourse following cerclage insertion should not be routinely recommended. Whilst routine serial sonographic **measurement of the cervix** is not recommended, it may be useful in individual cases following ultrasound-indicated cerclage to offer timely administration of **steroids** or **in utero transfer**.

Routine fetal **fibronectin testing** is not recommended post-cerclage. However, the high negative predictive value of fetal fibronectin testing for subsequent delivery at less than 30 weeks of gestation in asymptomatic high-risk women with a cerclage in place may provide reassurance to women and clinicians in individual cases.

When to Remove Cervical Cerclage

A transvaginal cervical cerclage should be electively removed before labour, usually at **37^{+0} weeks of gestation**, unless delivery is by elective Caesarean section, in which case suture removal could be delayed until this time. Elective removal is advisable owing to the potential risk of **cervical injury** in labour and the minimal risk to a neonate born at this gestation.

All women with a transabdominal cerclage require delivery by Caesarean section, and the abdominal suture may be left in place following delivery.

Further Reading

RCOG (2011). Cervical Cerclage. Green-top Guideline 60. Royal College of Obstetricians of Gynaecologists.

NICE guideline (2019). [NG25]. Preterm labour and birth (amended August 2019). www.nice.org.uk/guidance/ng25/resources/surveillance-report-exceptional-review-2017-preterm-labour-and-birth-2015-nice-guideline-ng25-4353994909/chapter/Surveillance-decision.

PART III

Gynaecology

11 Total Abdominal Hysterectomy

Abha Govind

Video Duration | 4 mins 47 secs

Overview

Abdominal hysterectomy is often the first major gynaecological procedure that trainees become competent in. Whilst laparoscopic hysterectomy may have gained popularity in recent years, the abdominal approach gives the trainee an understanding of pelvic anatomy and provides a basis from which he/she can progress to hysterectomy through the vaginal or laparoscopic routes.

Introduction

The number of total abdominal hysterectomies **(TAH)** for normal sized uteruses has fallen as a result of the efficacy of Mirena IUS in treating menstrual disorders. Where possible, women also desire less invasive and more cosmetic procedures and hence prefer to undergo laparoscopic or vaginal hysterectomy for a normal sized uterus. Many TAHs performed nowadays occur in women who have had previous operations such as Caesarean sections or have pelvic pathology; for example, endometriosis, adhesions and large uterine fibroids. Trainees therefore rarely have the opportunity to perform relatively uncomplicated TAH and this chapter discusses the basic steps and tips for the procedure.

Procedure

TAH is done through a **low transverse** or **Pfannenstiel** incision. The nature of the pathology, the size of the patient, previous operations and the mobility and size of the uterus to be removed may sometimes necessitate a **midline** approach.

There are enormous variations in style and technique for TAH. In training years, one should grasp the opportunity to watch and assist as many seniors as possible.

Empty the bladder using a Foley's **catheter** and clean the vagina using a swab on a sponge forceps. With the patient **supine** and with a **head-down tilt, prep** and **drape** the site of surgery. Most gynaecologists find it easiest to perform the procedure from the patient's **right side.**

How to Perform Operative Procedures in Obstetrics and Gynaecology, First Edition.
Edited by Wai Yoong, Abha Govind, and Wasim Lodhi.
© 2020 John Wiley & Sons Ltd. Published 2020 by John Wiley & Sons Ltd.
Companion website: www.wiley.com/go/yoong/obgyn

Incision

Most TAHs can be performed through a transverse suprapubic incision. **Palpate** the upper border of the symphysis pubis and make an incision **2–3 cm** above. If possible, try and make it below the upper limit of the pubic hairline, but it can be modified depending on the presence of a skin crease. Incise through **skin, superficial fascia** and **fat** down to the **rectus sheath.** The sheath is incised to reveal the vertical fibres of the **rectus abdominis,** 3 cm on either side of the midline. The **median raphe** and the underlying **pyramidalis muscles** are exposed. Hold the rectus sheath with your index and middle finger or Kocher or Littlewood tissue forceps to pull the tissue up under tension. Incise the median raphe until the pyramidalis falls away to expose the peritoneum. The incision can be further developed using index fingers of the two hands in both 'north–south' and 'east–west' direction in a **modified Cohen technique.** If this is a repeat procedure, sharp dissection using Mayo scissors will be needed. Be mindful of the **perforating vessels** when separating the rectus muscle from the sheath as well as the **inferior epigastric artery** or its branches, which run below the rectus abdominis muscle. Try to diathermise these before the incised ends retract into the muscle.

The peritoneum can be **picked up** with two Spencer-Wells forceps, felt between finger and thumb to ensure nothing is adherent to the back and then opened with scissors. With the peritoneum open, **sweep** a finger inside to check for adhesions and then **divide** the **peritoneum** initially in a cephalad direction and then inferiorly, looking for the translucent area which marks the fundus of the bladder.

When clinical circumstances – such as previous scars, enlarged fibroids or ovarian masses – require a **midline incision,** a lower midline incision is made first. This can be extended above and around the umbilicus if further access is needed. The subcutaneous tissue and fat are incised to reach the rectus sheath, which is subsequently opened in the upper part. The extraperitoneal fat between the two rectus abdominis muscles will be seen. The peritoneum is opened carefully as above.

The small bowel is **packed** using moist abdominal packs in order to displace this from the surgical field. A **self-retaining** Balfour **retractor** is introduced to improve access. The uterus is drawn out of the abdominal wound using the surgeon's nondominant hand and two straight heavy tissue forceps are placed at the cornual ends. If there is a large fibroid impairing the **delivery of the uterus,** a **myoma screw** in the bed of the uppermost myoma will allow traction. There are several versions of hysterectomy clamps (such as Gwilliams, Maingot and Roberts) and you will see them during your training.

The **round ligament** is clamped separately using a Spencer-Wells artery forceps and cut whilst it is held under tension by the assistant. This opens the two leaves of the **broad ligament.** Use the scissors to open the anterior leaf until the **utero-vesical fold** is reached (Figure 11.1). The **posterior leaf** of the broad ligament is pushed back with the index finger and the ureter can be seen and felt between the index finger and thumb at this stage. The **ureter** will be on the medial side and the great vessels of the pelvic side walls on the lateral side of the fingers. When rolled between finger and thumb the ureter feels firm, thick and incompressible. As it escapes from the grip, it gives a characteristic 'snap'. The posterior leaf of the broad ligament is incised using scissors and the ovarian or infundibulo-pelvic ligament is ready to be transected, depending on whether the ovaries are being conserved or removed.

If ovaries are being conserved, a curved clamp is placed medial to the ovary, over the **ovarian ligament** and the Fallopian tube, and the intervening tissue is cut through. The ovarian pedicle is transfixed and secured twice using 0 Vicryl, to achieve haemostasis.

If oophorectomy is planned, then the **infudibulo-pelvic ligament** is placed on a stretch and the pedicle similarly transected after clamping (Figure 11.2). Ensure that the clamp is close to the ovary so as not to inadvertently injure the ureter at this point. The round ligament and ovarian pedicles sutures can be held in a small artery forceps.

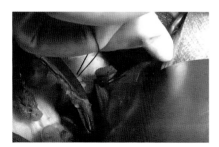

Figure 11.1 Opening the anterior leaf of the broad ligament.

The **bladder** is then reflected inferiorly. The anterior leaf of the broad ligament, is picked up with forceps and opened downwards and transversely with McIndoe scissors to open the loose fold of peritoneum forming the **utero-vesical** pouch (Figure 11.3). The bladder pillars are separated from the cervix and the bladder mobilised from the cervix using blunt dissection with a gauze swab wrapped around the index finger. Keep to the midline and avoid straying laterally in order to avoid injuring the bladder veins.

The **uterine arteries** can be secured with a curved clamp such as Gwilliams or Rogers near the junction of the body of the uterus with the cervix. These vessels are divided using a knife or scissors and the uterine pedicle is doubly ligated.

The next step is to divide the **parametrium** lateral to the cervix and it is good practice to **identify the ureter** in the ureteric canal of the parametrium by palpation between the finger and thumb of the right hand. The parametrium is clamped by applying traction to the fundus of the uterus over to one side (Figure 11.4). It is important to place the clamps immediately lateral to the wall of the cervix. The point of the clamp should be placed with great care, well away from the bladder and the ureter.

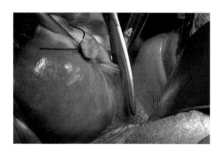

Figure 11.2 Securing the ovarian pedicle.

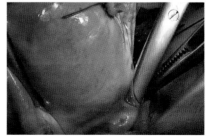

Figure 11.3 Separating the utero-vesical fold.

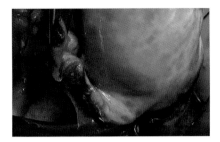

Figure 11.4 Clamping the parametrium.

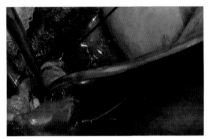

Figure 11.5 The vaginal cuff being held using Littlewood tissue forceps.

If the cervix is long, it may be necessary to place an additional clamp. This should always be placed medial to the previous pedicle. The space between the bladder and the vagina in the midline is relatively bloodless but the lateral vaginal plexus of veins together with the venous plexuses of the parametrium can bleed if traumatised.

The **vagina** can be finally **opened** anteriorly or posteriorly. If opened from the front, the anterior vaginal wall is first grasped in the midline with a Littlewood tissue forceps, after which it is incised with a knife. The opening is enlarged using the Mayo scissors. A curved Gwilliam clamp is placed on the **vaginal angle** and the tissue between the uterus and the clamp is cut through using scissors. The vaginal cuffs are then held using Littlewoods forceps (Figure 11.5).

The **vaginal angles** are ligated separately, and the vagina is usually closed using a continuous interlocking suture. Some surgeons leave the vagina open for drainage and oversew the edges to attain haemostasis.

Haemostasis of all pedicles is checked using a swab on a stick with pressure being placed for a minute if necessary. If there is a defined bleeding point, then it needs to be diathermised or sutured and haemostasis confirmed.

Closure

Closure of the pelvic or parietal peritoneum is not needed. A drain can be left in the pelvis or under the rectus sheath if needed and it can be brought out through the skin at a point inferior to the incision. The transverse abdominal incision is closed in **layers,** the rectus sheath approximated using 1 Vicryl and the skin closure using subcuticular 3–0 Vicryl suture.

Mass closure is the generally accepted method for midline closures using a loop nylon or PDS. The suture requires generous bites of tissue including the sheath, muscle and peritoneum.

Summary of Procedure Steps

- The patient is **supine** under **general anaesthesia.**
- The abdomen is **prepped** and **draped** and opened through a **Pfannensteil** incision. **Incise** the **skin, superficial fascia** and **fat.**
- Cut through **rectus sheath** and separate the muscle to expose the peritoneum.
- The uterus is exteriorised out of the incision.
- Clamp, cut and ligate the **round ligaments** to open the anterior leaf and push back the posterior leaf of the broad ligament.

- Clamp, cut and **ligate the ovarian ligament and tube** if ovaries are to be conserved. Include the infundibulopelvic ligament if oophorectomy is planned.
- Open the **utero-vesicle fold** of peritoneum and push the bladder down.
- The **uterine arteries** are secured and ligated on both sides.
- The **parametrium** is clamped and ligated on both sides.
- The bladder is pushed down and the **cervix is separated** from the **vagina** circumferentially.
- **Vaginal angles** are secured and vagina closed.

- Check **haemostasis in all pedicles.**
- Close the rectus sheath and apply **subcuticular absorbable** suture to the skin.

Further Reading

RCOG (May 2009). Consent advice no 4. Abdominal hysterectomy for benign conditions. www.rcog.org.uk/globalassets/documents/guidelines/consent-advice/ca4-15072010.pdf

Wells, E.C. (2008). Total abdominal hysterectomy and bilateral salpingo-oophorectomy. *Glob. libr. Women's Med.* https://doi.org/10.3843/GLOWM.10039.

12 Open Myomectomy

Abha Govind

Video Duration | 5 mins 23 secs

Overview

Myoma removal is most commonly done through the abdominal route but, depending on location, myomectomy can also be performed via the laparoscopic, vaginal or hysteroscopic approaches. In this chapter, the author discusses tips and techniques of open myomectomy.

Introduction

Open myomectomy is appropriate for many women with uterine fibroids. The surgeon's goal during **myomectomy** is to remove the myomas, reconstruct the uterus and preserve its function.

Indications

Myomectomy is indicated in women with **large uterine fibroids** who desire conservation of uterus. This surgery is indicated in women suffering from **severe anaemia, ureteral obstruction, lower limb venous thromboembolism, pelvic pressure** and **urinary retention** secondary to uterine fibroids.

Pre-operative Considerations

Prior to planning open myomectomy, accurate **assessment of the size, number and location** of the myomas is important. Although ultrasonography is adequate (**sonography** can differentiate fibroids from other pelvic pathology), magnetic resonance imaging (MRI) allows the best assessment of the size, number and location of the myomas. Women with myomas may have **anaemia** requiring correction before surgery. Women with multiple or large myomas may benefit from use of **cell salvage techniques** for autologous blood transfusion as this reduces the need for heterologous blood transfusion (which should also be available when undertaking surgery for large or multiple myomas).

The use of gonadotropin-releasing hormone (GnRH) agonists to decrease the size of the myomas enables the patient to improve their haemoglobin levels and also makes surgery technically easier.

Patients undergoing myomectomy should be **counselled** pre-operatively about the **risks** of haemorrhage and the small likelihood of proceeding to a

How to Perform Operative Procedures in Obstetrics and Gynaecology, First Edition.
Edited by Wai Yoong, Abha Govind, and Wasim Lodhi.
© 2020 John Wiley & Sons Ltd. Published 2020 by John Wiley & Sons Ltd.
Companion website: www.wiley.com/go/yoong/obgyn

hysterectomy. The patient must also be aware of the increased potential for **blood transfusion** intraoperatively and during recovery.

Abdominal Incision

The surgeon must first take into account the size and location of the myomas before deciding on the incision. With experience, even a large uterus with multiple myomas usually can be accessed through a **transverse lower abdominal incision**. Prior to reaching the lateral borders of the rectus abdominis, consider curving the fascial incision cephalad to avoid injury to the ileo-inguinal nerves. Detaching the midline linea alba from the anterior abdominal wall up to the umbilicus often improves access to the enlarged uterus. When the uterus is above the umbilicus and cannot be delivered through the transverse incision, a **vertical midline incision** would be more appropriate. A slight Trendelenburg position helps to ensure exposure.

Delivery of the uterus through the incision isolates the surgical field from the bowel, bladder and ureters, thus reducing the risk of injury. Judicious use of the myoma screw helps to facilitate delivery of uterus but the insertion point can bleed briskly on occasions. Ensure that the screw is inserted in the myoma to be removed and away from the normal myometrium and cornual end of the fallopian tubes. Once the delivered, **inspect and palpate** uterus for myomas. Identify the fundus and the virtual position of the uterine cavity by locating both cornua and imagining a straight line between them.

Managing Intraoperative Blood Loss

Vasopressin, tranexamic acid, misoprostol as well as application of uterine and ovarian vessel tourniquet have all been used to reduce intraoperative blood loss. They have different mechanisms of action. **Vasopressin** diluted in normal saline, injected below the vascular pseudo-capsule, causes vasoconstriction of capillaries. Intravascular injection should be avoided as rare cases of bradycardia and cardiovascular collapse have been reported. **Tranexamic acid** is an antifibrinolytic agent and can be given intravenously at the start of surgery. **Misoprostol** inserted vaginally two hours prior to surgery induces myometrial contraction and compression of the uterine vessels. Placement of a **tourniquet** around the lower uterine segment, including the infundibular pelvic ligaments, has also been used. Some surgeons incise the broad ligament bilaterally and pass the tourniquet through the broad ligament to avoid compromising blood flow to the ovaries. Always ensure that the tourniquet does not inadvertently encompass the fallopian tubes.

Uterine Incision

The preferred uterine incision is a vertical one on the anterior surface of the uterus. This minimises blood loss and prevents the ovaries from adhering to the posterior wall of the uterus postoperatively. It is often possible to remove multiple myomas through a **single incision** but multiple incisions are sometimes required. It is felt that the amount of peritoneal surface injury correlates with the extent of adhesion formation. Thus, minimising the length and number of the uterine incisions is a general strategy that should be adopted.

Myomas are encased within a **pseudo-capsule** and no distinct 'vascular pedicle' exists at its base. Incising through the pseudocapsule exposes the tissue planes, after which **blunt and sharp dissection** is used to enucleate the myoma out of the capsule (Figures 12.1 and 12.2). The surgeon can use a knife, Mayo scissors, electrocoagulation, laser or blunt dissection to accomplish this.

The myoma screw can be used to apply traction to or stabilise the fibroid so as to facilitate enucleation (Figure 12.3).

Small myomas not identified through sonography can be palpated and removed at the time of open surgery. **Tunnels** can be created within the myometrium to extract myomas that are distant from an incision and care must be taken to occlude any resultant dead space to avoid haematoma.

Myomectomy often leaves an **oozing cavitary defect** in the myometrium and **interrupted sutures** afford a greater chance of tissue approximation and **occlusion of dead space.** Layered interrupted sutures are time consuming but provide the best opportunity at tissue coaptation

(Figure 12.4). After the myometrial layers have been adequately repaired, excess redundant serosa is 'trimmed' and the serosal defect repaired with a fine polyglycolic suture in a running 'baseball mitt' fashion (Figure 12.5). This allows a minimum of exposed suture material and decreases adhesion formation. Use of ADEPT® (4% ICODEXTRIN) (BAXTER) solution or similar **adhesion barriers** may help limit adhesion formation. The tourniquet is then released and the surgical site carefully inspected for bleeding. The abdominal incision is closed routinely.

Complications of Myomectomy

Open myomectomy may be complicated by haemorrhage, infection, bowel obstruction, adhesion formation, injury to bowel,

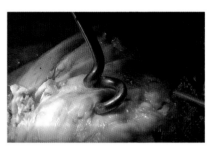

Figure 12.3 A myoma screw can be used to stabilise the fibroid so as to facilitate enucleation.

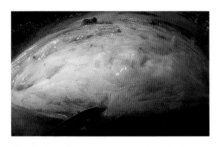

Figure 12.1 The pseudocapsule is incised to expose the myoma.

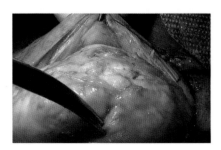

Figure 12.2 The myoma is enucleated using sharp and blunt dissection.

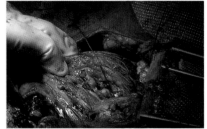

Figure 12.4 The myometrium is repaired in layers, ensuring that any dead space is obliterated.

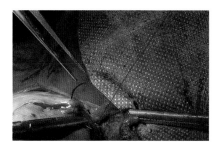

Figure 12.5 The serosa is repaired using a 'baseball mitt' technique.

bladder, fallopian tubes and ureter, as well as wound dehiscence. Furthermore, 20–25% of patients undergoing myomectomy may require a second operation, usually hysterectomy, because of recurrence of symptoms. Although extremely rare, uncontrolled intraoperative haemorrhage may lead to a **hysterectomy.** If the cavity is breached during myomectomy, patients must be advised that an elective **Caesarean section is necessary in subsequent pregnancies** to prevent uterine rupture during labour.

Postoperative **febrile morbidity** can occur, and it is often difficult to distinguish infection from pyrexia caused by prostaglandin release during myomectomy.

A significant but not easily quantified sequelae of myomectomy **is subfertility** caused by the procedure. Subsequent **adhesion formation** may cause tubal occlusion as well as decrease the ability of the fimbria to pick up an oocyte.

Further Reading

McIlveen, M. and Li, T.C. (2005). Myomectomy: a review of surgical technique. *Hum. Fertil. (Camb.)* 8 (1): 27–33. PMID: 15823848.

Saridogan, E. (2016). Surgical treatment of fibroids in heavy menstrual bleeding. *Womens Health (Lond.)* 12 (1): 53–62. PMID: 26693796.

13 Hysteroscopic Resection of Fibroids

Sayantana Das and Wasim Lodhi

Video Duration | 3 mins 25 secs

Overview

The authors share tips on how to assemble the operative hysteroscope and the technique of transcervical resection of fibroids.

Introduction

Operative hysteroscopy now forms part of standard gynaecological practice. It is **minimally invasive** and involves an endoscopic optical lens being inserted through the cervix to diagnose and treat various types of intrauterine pathology. It is also diagnostic and a treatment tool for abnormal uterine bleeding. Endoscopic technology has been rapidly developing since the introduction of **distention medium** around 30 years ago. Present day smaller diameter hysteroscopes have allowed operative hysteroscopy to become a predominately **office-based** procedure.

Indications for Operative Hysteroscopy Include

1 Resection of submucosal fibroids.
2 Removal of endometrial polyps.
3 Division of uterine septum.
4 Intrauterine adhesiolysis.
5 Removal of foreign body.

This chapter will focus on transcervical resection of fibroids **(TCRF)**, which is a method of excising submucous uterine fibroids, which can cause heavy menstrual bleeding, recurrent miscarriages or subfertility. TCRF is usually performed under a general anaesthetic.

Classification systems have been devised to enable accurate description of submucous fibroids and assist clinicians in determining the likelihood of successful hysteroscopic surgery. The most widely used classification is that adopted by the European Society of Gynaecological Endoscopy (ESGE). Grade 0 and Grade 1 fibroids can be easily removed hysteroscopically but Grade 2 fibroids (>50% of fibroid is in the myometrium) are not suitable for transcervical resection.

How to Perform Operative Procedures in Obstetrics and Gynaecology, First Edition.
Edited by Wai Yoong, Abha Govind, and Wasim Lodhi.
© 2020 John Wiley & Sons Ltd. Published 2020 by John Wiley & Sons Ltd.
Companion website: www.wiley.com/go/yoong/obgyn

Instruments for Hysteroscopic Resection

1 Hysteroscopes may be classified as **rigid** or **flexible; operative hysteroscopes** are predominantly **rigid**.

2 The **telescope** has three parts: eye piece, barrel and objective lens. They are available in various angles (commonly 0° or 30°).

3 Light source.

4 Stack.

5 Sheath:
Diagnostic 4–5 mm (smaller sizes are also available)
Operative 7–10 mm.

6 **Distending medium**:
Diagnostic – CO2/normal saline
Operative – Normal saline/glycine.

7 Dilator set.

Assembly of Resectoscope

1 The resectoscope is a specialised electrosurgical (monopolar or bipolar) endoscope which consists of an inner sheath and outer sheath.

2 The **outer sheath** is for fluid distention.

3 The inner sheath has a common channel for the telescope fluid medium and electrode.

4 The **inner sheath** is inserted into the outer one and the two are locked by aligning them (Figure 13.1).

5 The double armed electrode is fitted to a **trigger device** that pushes the electrode out beyond the sheath and then retracts it back within.

6 The hysteroscope is introduced into the working element and a click can be heard as it is secured in place. Most resectoscopes have **30° telescopes,** with the lens angled towards the electrode to permit a clear view of the near operative field.

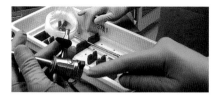

Figure 13.1 Aligning the inner and outer sheaths.

7 The operator's index finger is usually placed in the trigger and this ensures that the resecting loop slides freely within the combined unit.

8 The cutting loop electrode is used to resect submucous myomas.

Distending Medium for Operative Hysteroscopy

Normal saline (0.9% NaCl) is safe and usually available in 3 Litre bags delivered using an infusion pump system such as Hamou Endomat. Normal saline is not suitable for monopolar electrosurgery as saline is an efficient conductor of electrons and does not permit a current density that is high enough for tissue action. When fluid deficit exceeds 1 L, the surgeon has to be vigilant for excessive vascular absorption leading to fluid overload and pulmonary oedema. Glycine, which is a hypo-osmolar solution, is used with monopolar devices. Fluid overload is likely but can produce hyponatraemia which can lead to life-threatening cerebral oedema.

Procedure

The patient is placed in the lithotomy position and a bimanual pelvic examination conducted to determine uterine size, mobility and position. Prior to starting, ensure that the hysteroscope assembly and outflow/inflow tubes are correctly connected; the light lead and camera are attached to the telescope and white balance undertaken; and verify that the correct distension medium is used before turning on the automated pump delivery system.

The cervix is visualised with a bivalve speculum or Sims retractor and a tenaculum is applied to the anterior cervical lip. The uterus is sounded to establish its length and the cervix is dilated to 1 mm more than the diameter of the resectoscope. In most cases, cervical dilation up to Hegar 9 should suffice for the insertion of a standard size operating hysteroscope.

Ideally, an electronic pressure-controlled suction/irrigation pump such as Hamou Endomat Irrigation System (Karl Stortz) is used to deliver fluid under pressure, but a manual hand-inflated pressure bag is equally adequate. The operative hysteroscope is placed in the external os and is inserted under direct visualisation, with distension medium flowing. It is imperative that the irrigation inflow remains open and the outflow valve closed (Figure 13.2): this maintains an intrauterine pressure sufficient for visualising the endometrial cavity. Inspect both tubal ostia by rotating the light lead. Any operating instruments should be under direct vision so that any uterine injury is identified.

The loop of the resectoscope is then extended to the most distant portion of the myoma, and current is applied as the resectoscope is withdrawn towards the operator (Figure 13.3). It is important for the surgeon to resect towards and not away from him or herself. A grasping forceps and curette can be used to remove resected tissue.

Tips and Trouble-Shooting Points

1 If the visualisation field is cloudy, the outflow valve can be intermittently opened and closed to flush out any residue or blood. The outflow valve can be left partially open to allow for fluid circulation if necessary.

2 Avoid touching the intrauterine walls as this can cause contact bleeding, which will obscure the field.

3 Check the fluid deficit – a fluid deficit of >1000 ml warrants re-evaluation of whether the procedure should continue.

4 At the end of the procedure, always calculate and record the fluid deficit.

5 Medical debulking two to three months prior to resection, using a gonadotrophin releasing hormone analogue (such as goserelin) can help shrink a large fibroid by up to 50%.

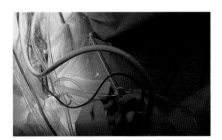

Figure 13.2 Controlling irrigation and suction outflow valves.

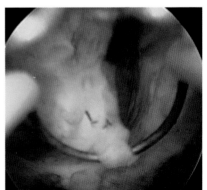

Figure 13.3 Resection is always performed towards the surgeon.

6 For large myomas, a two-stage surgical procedure should be discussed. After the first TCRF, a second procedure can be contemplated in three months if symptoms persist.

Further Reading

Wamsteker, K., Emanuel, M.H., and de Kruif, J.H. (1993). Transcervical hysteroscopic resection of submucous fibroids for abnormal uterine bleeding: results regarding the degree of intramural extension. *Obstet. Gynecol.* 82: 736–740.

Younas, K., Hadoura, E., Majoko, F., and Bunkheila, A. (2016). A review of evidence-based management of uterine fibroids. *Obstet. Gynaecol.* 18: 33–42.

14 Diagnostic Laparoscopy

Charlotte Austen and Abha Govind

Video Duration | 10 mins 25 secs

Overview

Diagnostic laparoscopy is a mandatory clinical competency for the gynaecology trainee. Familiarity with the equipment and instruments as well as technical competence with Verres needle insertion and trocar and port placements are crucial for the practising gynaecologist.

Introduction

In this chapter, the authors explain the closed Verres entry technique and how to insert and remove ports. The important role of the assistant in bladder catheterisation and uterine manipulation is also covered.

The Stack System

The stack system is the **control centre** for the laparoscopic procedure. The high definition camera, primary monitor screen, carbon dioxide insufflator, light source and digital printer are all connected to the main stack.

The 'Bottom End' Preparation and Patient Position

For gynaecological laparoscopies, it is often necessary to manipulate the uterus in order to get better views of pelvic anatomy and to improve ergonomics during operative laparoscopy. The vulva, vagina and abdomen are cleaned and draped. The bladder is emptied with an in-out **catheter.** The vagina and cervix are visualised using a **Sim's** speculum and the cervix grasped with a tenaculum or **vulsellum.** A **Spackman cannula** is inserted into the uterine cavity and used to antevert and retrovert the uterus. It is sometimes necessary to serially **dilate** the cervix to allow the Spackman cannula insertion for **uterine manipulation.** The Sims **speculum** is then **removed** and the legs lowered and adducted.

At the start of the procedure, the operating table should be horizontal, and the patient initially lies prone with her legs in

How to Perform Operative Procedures in Obstetrics and Gynaecology, First Edition.
Edited by Wai Yoong, Abha Govind, and Wasim Lodhi.
© 2020 John Wiley & Sons Ltd. Published 2020 by John Wiley & Sons Ltd.
Companion website: www.wiley.com/go/yoong/obgyn

lithotomy position on a non-slip mattress. When CO_2 insufflation is complete, the **Trendelenberg** tilt is employed: this uses gravity to move viscera caudally, thus facilitating visual access to pelvic organs. Trendelenburg position was originally described as the torso supine and the legs upon the shoulders of an assistant; however, the term is now used to describe any head-down position – classically a 45° head-down tilt.

Laparoscopic Techniques

The patient's abdomen is cleaned and draped. The **insufflator tubing** is connected to the CO2 supply and the **light lead** to the light source. The **Veress** needle is then tested for **patency** and baseline flow rate. The **laparoscope** can either be **5 mm** or **10 mm** in diameter and either 0° or 30° depending on surgeon preference and the procedure undertaken. The initial incision needs to allow for the relevant **sized primary port** and laparoscope.

Primary Veress Insertion

The **abdomen** is **palpated** to check for any masses before insertion of the Veress needle. If there is minimal concern about intra-abdominal adhesions, an intra-**umbilical** primary incision can be made. This site is the **thinnest** and the **least vascular area** with a **fixed peritoneum** and has the advantage of being **cosmetic.** The primary incision for laparoscopy should be **vertical** from the **base of the umbilicus** (not in the skin below the umbilicus). Care should be taken not to incise so deeply as to enter the peritoneal cavity.

Palmer's point (2–3 cm below the **costal margin** in the **midclavicular line**) should be considered if there is likelihood of **adhesions** (Figure 14.3).

Using a Veress needle for primary entry into the abdomen is the most common insufflation method in gynaecological surgery, whereas most general surgeons use the **Hasson's entry** method as an alternative.

Once the initial incision is made, the **Veress needle** is held in a pen grip and gently inserted at **90°** to the skin through the initial incision (Figure 14.1). **Two clicks** can be felt and heard, corresponding to entry through the **rectus sheath** and **parietal peritoneum respectively. Palmer's test** is then used to confirm correct intra-peritoneal position of the Veress needle – a drop of **saline** placed on the Veress will be sucked in due to the **negative** intra-abdominal **pressure**. A fluid **aspiration** test can also be done using a 10 ml syringe and this should not contain bowel contents. Excessive lateral movement of the needle must be avoided as this may convert a small Veress injury in the wall of the bowel or vessel into a complex tear.

The gas tubing is then attached to the Veress needle. The most predictive test for correct intraperitoneal placement of the Veress needle is that the initial insufflation pressure remains low (<8 mmHg) and gas is flowing freely (BSGE/RCOG 2008). During insufflation, the **set pressure** can be increased to **20–25 mmHg** and uniform abdominal distension can be seen with

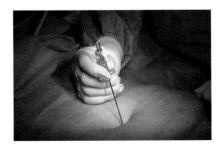

Figure 14.1   Using a pen grip to insert the Veress needle.

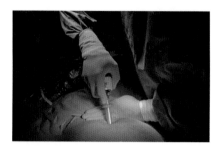

Figure 14.2 'Palming' the primary trocar with the index finger on the shaft.

accompanying loss of liver dullness on percussion. The umbilical incision is then extended with a blade to allow insertion of the primary trocar (5 or 10 mm). The **primary trocar** is held in the palm, with the **index finger** against the shaft to prevent over insertion (Figure 14.2). The trocar is inserted at a 45° angle to the skin, using the non-dominant hand to splint the upper abdomen. This is then removed and the camera inserted through the retaining sleeve. Once intraperitoneal access is confirmed visually, the patient position is converted to a Trendelenburg tilt to facilitate access to pelvic organs. A **360° surveillance** of the pelvis and upper abdomen must be performed.

Insertion of Secondary Port/s

The **secondary ports** are inserted next, using the **obliterated umbilical artery** as the landmark in order to avoid the **inferior epigastric vessels,** which lie just medially. **Transillumination** helps to identify superficial skin vessels and the secondary ports are inserted under direct vision **perpendicular to** the **skin.** Once the peritoneum is 'tented' by the trocar, it is then **angled towards** the **pelvis** to avoid injury to the bowel. An additional secondary port can be inserted under direct vision on the contralateral side if required. An inadvertent

injury from a secondary port entry could be considered negligent. Once all the ports are in place, the **set insufflation** pressure can be reduced to 12–15 mmHg to maintain pneumoperitoneum.

Exit Techniques

On completion of the procedure, check by direct visualisation that there has not been a 'through-and-through' injury of bowel adherent under the umbilicus.

All **ports** must be **removed under** direct **vision,** and any remaining gas expelled. **Midline ports >10 mm** and lateral ports **>7 mm** must have the rectus sheath closed using a **J needle** to prevent port site hernia or dehiscence (Figure 14.4).

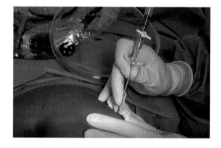

Figure 14.3 Insufflation at Palmer's point.

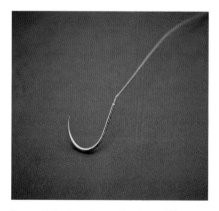

Figure 14.4 J needle used to close midline ports >10 mm.

The skin incisions can be closed with absorbable sutures or tissue glue. The Spackman can be removed from the uterus and the vulsellum from the cervix.

Complications

The commonest problem with the Veress technique is failed entry. Closed entry can cause bowel (1 : 1000) and vascular injury especially if adhesions are present. Rarely retroperitoneal haemorrhage, bladder injury and injury to over distended stomach can occur.

Further Reading

BSGE/RCOG (2008). Green-top Guideline no 49. Preventing Entry-related Gynaecological Laparoscopic Injuries.

RCOG (2017). Diagnostic Laparoscopy (Consent Advice No. 2). Royal College of Obstetricians and Gynaecologists. www.rcog.org.uk/ guidelines-research-services/guidelines/ consent-advice-2.

15 Operative Laparoscopy

Charlotte Austen and Abha Govind

Video Duration | 6 mins 24 secs

Overview

This chapter explains the basic techniques for the more common laparoscopic procedures such as adhesiolysis, ovarian drilling and ovarian cystectomy.

Introduction

The laparoscopic approach is the optimal way of performing adhesiolysis and ovarian cystectomy as this is associated with smaller incisions, less pain and bleeding as well as a more rapid recovery.

Adhesiolysis

Adhesions are fibrous bands of scar tissue, often resulting from previous surgery. They form between internal viscus and tissues, joining them together in an abnormal fashion. **Laparoscopic adhesiolysis** is an effective management option for patients with adhesions presenting with chronic abdominal pain, bowel obstruction or subfertility.

Adhesions can be lysed with sharp or blunt **dissection,** and with or without a power source. It is important to maintain **haemostasis** and an energy source, such as laparoscopic **bipolar** forceps or a

Harmonic scalpel (Ethicon) is often used. When using an energy source, it is critical that both blades are constantly in vision and that 'hot' adhesions are not dropped directly onto the underlying bowel as this could cause a **thermal injury.** When performing adhesiolysis, adhesions should be held under tension, either by gravity or by using laparoscopic **graspers** to allow for ease of cutting (Figure 15.1). Slow dissection is safer as it allows direct vision of what is being dissected.

Top Tips

- Inspect the pelvic cavity prior to beginning adhesiolysis.
- Grasp adhesions from the side contralateral to where you plan to make the first cut.
- Divide superficial adhesions first to ensure unimpeded access to deeper ones in case bleeding occurs.

How to Perform Operative Procedures in Obstetrics and Gynaecology, First Edition.
Edited by Wai Yoong, Abha Govind, and Wasim Lodhi.
© 2020 John Wiley & Sons Ltd. Published 2020 by John Wiley & Sons Ltd.
Companion website: www.wiley.com/go/yoong/obgyn

- Coagulate thick or vascular adhesions with bipolar diathermy prior to division.
- Cut adhesions at both ends and remove the tissue rather than just dividing it.

Ovarian Drilling

Laparoscopic **ovarian drilling** is a technique used in the treatment of anovulatory subfertility in women with polycystic ovaries (Figure 15.2). The procedure can trigger ovulation in women who have **polycystic ovary syndrome** (PCOS). Successful ovarian drilling avoids the risks of ovarian hyperstimulation syndrome and multiple pregnancies seen with the use of gonadotrophins. **Standardisation** of this surgical technique is **lacking.** The procedure is often performed with an insulated unipolar needle electrode with a non-insulated distal end measuring

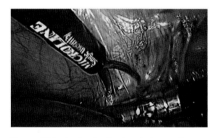

Figure 15.1 Lysis of adhesions between the small bowel and anterior abdominal wall. Note both blades of the scissors are seen, and the grasper is used to stretch the adhesions in order to facilitate cutting.

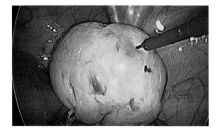

Figure 15.2 Laparoscopic ovarian drilling using unipolar needle electrode.

1–2 cm. The **number of punctures** is empirically chosen depending on the ovarian size. In the original procedure, 3–8 diathermy punctures (each of 3 mm diameter and 2–4 mm depth) per ovary were applied, using a power setting of 200–300 W for 2–4 seconds. (Gjönnaess 1984). Most surgeons perform **four punctures** per ovary, each for 4 seconds at 40 W ('rule of 4'), delivering 640 J of energy per ovary (the lowest effective dose recommended) (Armar et al. 1990).

Ovarian Cystectomy

Large, persistent or **symptomatic** ovarian cysts usually need to be surgically removed. Surgery is also recommended if there are concerns that the cyst could be **cancerous.** Most cysts can be removed using **laparoscopy.** If the cyst is particularly **large,** or if there is suspicion of malignancy, a **laparotomy** may be recommended. A serum **CA-125** assay does not need to be undertaken in all premenopausal women with simple cysts. Lactate dehydrogenase (LDH), α-FP and hCG should be measured in all women under 40 years of age with a complex ovarian mass because of the possibility of germ cell tumours. A **transvaginal ultrasonography** is preferable due to its increased sensitivity to diagnose ovarian cysts. The laparoscopic approach for management of ovarian masses that are presumed to be benign is associated with **lower postoperative morbidity** and **shorter recovery time** and is preferred to laparotomy in suitable patients. **Spillage** of cyst contents should be **avoided** where possible as preoperative and intraoperative assessment cannot absolutely preclude malignancy. Consideration should be given to the use of an endoscopic bag in order to avoid peritoneal spill of cystic contents as malignancy cannot be excluded until the specimen is sent for histology.

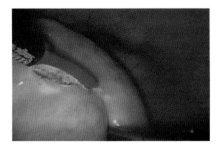

Figure 15.3 Incision in the capsule of the ovarian cyst using monopolar scissors.

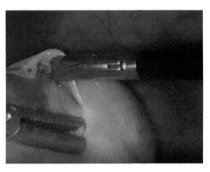

Figure 15.4 'Grasp and peel' technique using two graspers.

Laparoscopic ovarian cystectomy is usually performed using the 'grasp and peel' technique. An initial 1 cm incision is made in the ovarian **capsule** with an energy device; typically, a **monopolar laparoscopic hook** or scissors (Figure 15.3). This incision is then enlarged using sharp and blunt dissection. The apex of the incision edges is grasped with **toothed graspers** and pulled in opposite directions (Figure 15.4). The cyst wall is gently peeled away from the ovarian cortex, with monopolar or bipolar energy being used for haemostasis. Once the cyst is removed from the ovary, it can be placed in an **endoscopic bag** and decompressed for removal. Any bleeding areas on the ovary can be treated using **bipolar diathermy**.

Further Reading

Armar, N.A., McGarrigle, H.H., Honour, J. et al. (1990). Laparoscopic ovarian diathermy in the management of anovulatory infertility in women with polycystic ovaries: endocrine changes and clinical outcome. *Fertil. Steril.* 53 (1): 45–49. PubMed PMID: 2136836.

Gjönnaess, H. (1984). Polycystic ovarian syndrome treated by ovarian electrocautery through the laparoscope. *Fertil. Steril.* 41 (1): 20–25. PubMed PMID: 6692959.

RCOG (2011). Management of suspected ovarian masses in premenopausal women. Greentop Guideline No. 62. RCOG/BSGE Joint Guideline November 2011. www.rcog.org.uk/globalassets/documents/guidelines/gtg_62.pdf.

16 Laparoscopic Salpingectomy for Ectopic Pregnancy

Wasim Lodhi

Video Duration | 6 mins 25 secs

Overview

Surgical competence in the laparoscopic management of ectopic pregnancy is now an essential component of gynaecological training. This chapter provides important technical tips on laparoscopic salpingectomy, in this case using an endoscopic loop.

Introduction

With high resolution transvaginal sonography, serum β-HCG assay and increased vigilance, cases of ectopic pregnancy are being diagnosed earlier. A laparoscopic surgical approach is preferable to an open one as the former is associated with a more cosmetic incision, less pain and a quicker recovery. In the presence of a healthy contralateral tube, salpingectomy should be performed in preference to salpingotomy (Elson et al. 2016).

Laparoscopic Salpingectomy

Salpingectomy can be performed by using electrocautery (**bipolar diathermy forceps**) to the mesosalpinx followed by incision along the mesosalpinx and across the proximal tube using laparoscopic scissors. The **Harmonic scalpel** is a surgical instrument used to simultaneously cut and cauterise tissue. Unlike electrosurgery, the Harmonic scalpel uses ultrasonic vibrations to cut and cauterise tissue instead of electric current.

Laparoscopic Salpingostomy

In women with a history of fertility-reducing factors (previous ectopic pregnancy, contralateral tubal damage, previous abdominal surgery, previous pelvic inflammatory disease), salpingotomy should be considered (Elson et al. 2016). If so, women should be informed about the risk of persistent

How to Perform Operative Procedures in Obstetrics and Gynaecology, First Edition.
Edited by Wai Yoong, Abha Govind, and Wasim Lodhi.
© 2020 John Wiley & Sons Ltd. Published 2020 by John Wiley & Sons Ltd.
Companion website: www.wiley.com/go/yoong/obgyn

trophoblast with the need for serum β-HCG level follow-up. They should also be counselled of the small risk that they may need further treatment in the form of systemic methotrexate or salpingectomy.

For **salpingostomy,** a linear incision is made on the most prominent and distended antimesenteric border of the fallopian tube with a **monopolar hook or scissors.** Products of conception are separated and flushed using irrigation fluid under pressure and aspirated out. The tubal incision is left open and allowed to heal by secondary intention.

Ten Easy Steps to Perform a Laparoscopic Salpingectomy Using an Endoloop

Here we describe the laparoscopic salpingectomy procedure using an Endoloop (Ethicon).

1 Place the patient in modified Lloyd Davies position, clean and drape.
2 Perform **diagnostic laparoscopy** to confirm the findings.
3 Insert lateral ports under direct vision. Consider using a **10 mm trochar** on the **same side** as the ectopic pregnancy for easier retrieval of the fallopian tube once excised.
4 Use a **non-traumatic grasper** to manipulate the tube from the contralateral side; for example, for a right-sided ectopic pregnancy it is easier to manipulate the fallopian tube by introducing the grasper from the left port.
5 If there is blood in the peritoneal cavity, **suction irrigation is performed.** This will improve the brightness and resolution of the screen images.
6 Introduce the Endoloop through the port on the ipsilateral (same) side as the ectopic pregnancy, taking care to keep

the tip of the Endoloop pointing upwards and bringing the loop over the affected fallopian tube (Figure 16.1). **Avoid getting** the loop **wet** as this will cause it to temporarily adhere to peritoneal viscera and will thus be more difficult to manipulate.

7 **Lay the Endoloop around the ectopic pregnancy and grasp** the ectopic pregnancy through the loop. The ectopic pregnancy is then carefully lifted through the loop (Figure 16.2).
8 The Endoloop is gently **tightened** by **snapping** the **distal end** of the plastic introducer. The position of the tightened Endoloop is carefully checked around the fallopian tube, ensuring that the ovary is not inadvertently caught in the pedicle. Use the plastic tip of Endoloop to **manipulate** and adjust the **position of** the **loop,** taking care not to tighten the loop before confirming the placement. The Endoloop is

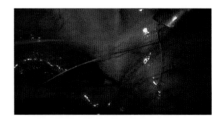

Figure 16.1 The Endoloop is placed over the ectopic pregnancy.

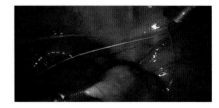

Figure 16.2 The ectopic pregnancy is lifted through the loop using endoscopic graspers.

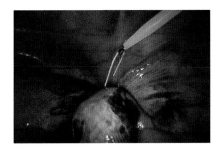

Figure 16.3 The Endoloop is tightened with the knot is directed towards the ectopic pregnancy.

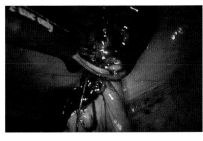

Figure 16.5 The ectopic pregnancy is cut using endoscopic scissors.

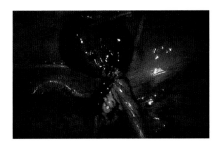

Figure 16.4 The knot is now secure, always confirm that the ovary is not inadvertently ligated.

then tightened ensuring that the **knot** is directed towards the ectopic pregnancy (Figure 16.3). The **thread is cut** using the **laparoscopic scissors** introduced through the contralateral port (Figure 16.4). A **second** Endoloop can be applied in a similar way to **doubly secure** the **pedicle.**

9 The **ectopic pregnancy** is held with a grasper through the ipsilateral side port

and **excised** with the laparoscopic scissors introduced through the contralateral port (Figure 16.5). The ectopic pregnancy can be removed either directly through the 10 mm port or by using an endoscopic specimen **retrieval bag** (Endobag/Endo Catch Medtronic (UK)) through the 10 mm port.

10 Confirm **haemostasis,** perform suction irrigation if needed and remove the lateral ports under direct vision. Release the gas and remove the primary port and suture the rectus sheath with a Vicryl **port closure needle** by Ethicon (J needle).

Further Reading

Elson, C.J., Salim, R., Potdar, N. et al. (2016). Diagnosis and management of ectopic pregnancy. *BJOG* 123: e15–e55. (Green-top Guideline No. 21 RCOG/AEPU Joint Guideline | November 2016).

17 Surgery for Vagina Prolapse Using Native Tissue

Wai Yoong

Video Duration | 7 mins 27 secs

Overview

This chapter highlights steps for anterior colporrhaphy and enterocele repair using native tissue. More complex surgery for recurrent prolapse such as sacrospinous fixation, sacrocolpopexy or laparoscopic repairs are beyond the scope of this chapter.

Introduction

Pelvic organ prolapse affects approximately 1 in 12 women in the United Kingdom (Cooper et al. 2015) and surgical repair of cystocele and recto-enterocele should form part of the repertoire of a gynaecologist. Primary repair of vaginal prolapse is performed using native tissue and two simple techniques to restore anatomy are described. The reader should refer to the video chapter to get better understanding of the techniques.

Anterior Colporrhaphy

The patient is first placed in the lithotomy position with her buttocks 1–2 cm slightly overhanging the operating bed. A **Lone Star retractor (Cooper Surgicals)** can be used to hold back the vulva and facilitate vaginal access. The skin over the cystocele is held under tension transversely using Allis tissue forceps. A solution of 20 ml of bupivacaine 0.5% w/v and adrenaline 1 : 200 000 is injected circumferentially to obtain tissue separation prior to incision.

A **full thickness skin incision** is made transversely exposing the cystocele and endopelvic fascia. The skin is mobilised from the prolapse using a combination of blunt and sharp dissection. The **cystocele** is held using a **Babcock forceps** and countertraction applied by holding the vaginal skin (Figure 17.1). Tissue planes can then be **separated by gently inserting a McIndoe scissors** and spreading its blades, thus mobilising the bladder from vaginal skin (Figure 17.2). Depending on the size of the cystocele, two or three buttressing sutures

How to Perform Operative Procedures in Obstetrics and Gynaecology, First Edition.
Edited by Wai Yoong, Abha Govind, and Wasim Lodhi.
© 2020 John Wiley & Sons Ltd. Published 2020 by John Wiley & Sons Ltd.
Companion website: www.wiley.com/go/yoong/obgyn

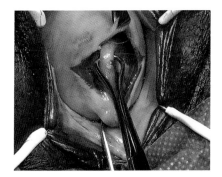

Figure 17.1 Full skin thickness incision exposing cystocele and endopelvic fascia.

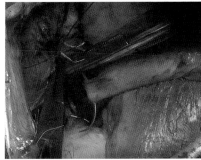

Figure 17.3 Endopelvic fascia reconstructed using buttressing sutures.

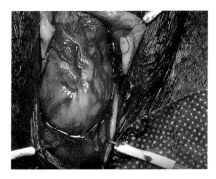

Figure 17.2 Cystocele mobilised from vaginal skin.

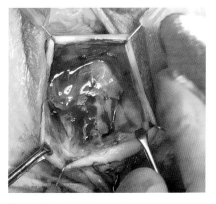

Figure 17.4 Full thickness incision posteriorly to expose enterocele and recto-vaginal septum.

are placed laterally (Figure 17.3). The cystocele is reduced using the Babcock forceps to approximately its original position. The sutures are then tightened to reconstruct the endopelvic fascia and lift the cystocele to its pre-prolapse anatomy.

Repair of Recto-Enterocele

The skin over the **recto-enterocele** is held taut using **Allis tissue forceps** and 20 ml of bupivacaine 0.5% w/v and adrenaline 1 : 200 000 is injected to produce vasoconstriction and hydrodissection of the tissue planes.

A **full thickness skin incision** is made transversely, exposing the prolapse and the **rectovaginal septum** (Figure 17.4). The vaginal skin is mobilised from the prolapse using a combination of blunt and sharp dissection. An enterocele is essentially a true hernia and the **avulsed recto-vaginal septum remnant** can be usually identified and held using Allis tissue forceps (Figure 17.5). The prolapse is held using a Babcock forceps and **recto-vaginal septum** further mobilised and developed (Figure 17.6). The recto-vaginal septum is then reattached to its origin using a **Mayo needle and interrupted PDS** (Figure 17.7). Redundant vaginal skin is excised and vagina reconstructed using Vicryl Rapide.

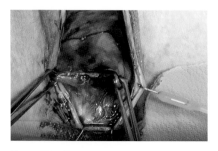

Figure 17.5 Recto-vaginal septum remnant held using Allis tissue forceps. The enterocele is visible above the septum remnant.

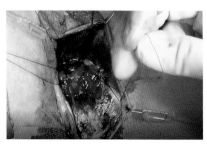

Figure 17.7 Prolapse reduced by reattaching recto-vaginal septum to its origin using Mayo needle and PDS.

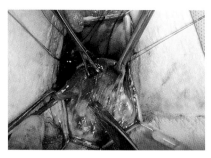

Figure 17.6 Recto-vaginal septum mobilised from the vaginal skin.

Further Reading

Cooper, J., Annappa, M., Dracocardos, D. et al. (2015). Prevalence of genital prolapse symptoms in primary care: a cross-sectional survey. *Int. Urogynecol. J.* 26 (4): 505–510.

NICE (2019). Urinary incontinence and pelvic organ prolapse in women: management [NG123]. Published: April 2019. www.nice.org.uk/guidance/ng123/chapter/Context.

18 Vaginal Hysterectomy for Prolapse

Jane Ding and Wai Yoong

> **Video Duration** 7 mins 32 secs

Overview

Vaginal hysterectomy is a very satisfying procedure to perform as it utilises a natural orifice to remove the female reproductive system, thus avoiding an abdominal incision. Whilst commonly indicated for uterine prolapse, this minimal invasive approach is recommended by the American College of Obstetricians and Gynecologists, as well as Cochrane Review as the gold standard for the removal of the uterus for benign disease. In this chapter, the authors describe the Heaney technique of vaginal hysterectomy for uterine prolapse.

Introduction

Traditionally, the main indications for vaginal hysterectomy are **uterine prolapse** and **heavy menstrual bleeding.** It is more advantageous to perform hysterectomy through the vaginal route for benign diseases as it results in no abdominal wound, less postoperative pain, earlier mobilisation and a shorter length of hospital stay. With the adoption of **Enhanced Recovery** pathways, it is now possible to perform vaginal hysterectomies as day cases. The principles of vaginal hysterectomy are similar to those of abdominal hysterectomy, with the steps performed in reversed order (Heaney technique).

Relative contraindications for vaginal hysterectomy:

- Uterine size larger than 12 week pregnancy with or without fibroids and ovarian pathology.
- Endometriosis or pelvic inflammatory disease.
- Previous Caesarean section/s.
- Malignant disease.
- Long narrow vagina.

Procedure

Vaginal hysterectomy can be performed under **general anaesthesia** or **regional anaesthesia.** The patient is placed in **lithotomy** position, with the **hips slightly hyperflexed.**

How to Perform Operative Procedures in Obstetrics and Gynaecology, First Edition.
Edited by Wai Yoong, Abha Govind, and Wasim Lodhi.
© 2020 John Wiley & Sons Ltd. Published 2020 by John Wiley & Sons Ltd.
Companion website: www.wiley.com/go/yoong/obgyn

Intraoperative prophylactic antibiotics are normally given. An indwelling Foley catheter is inserted. Bimanual examination is performed to assess uterine size, mobility and descent. A vaginal surgery tray is attached as an extension below the table for placement of instruments. Different types of retractors can be used to improve visualisation, and in the video footage a **Lone Star retractor (Cooper Surgicals)** is used and can be seen in the figures.

Grasp the cervix with two **Vulsellum tissue forceps** for traction. Infiltrate the subepithelial tissue with a solution of 20 ml of bupivacaine 0.5% w/v and adrenaline 1 : 200 000 circumferentially at 2–3 cm caudal to the cervical os. This helps **develop tissue planes** and reduce perioperative bleeding.

Incise the vaginal mucosa **circumferentially** at the level of infiltration and ensure that **full skin thickness** is achieved so that the cervix is reached. Applying downward traction on the cervix, the **bladder is held with Babcock forceps,** whilst the cervico-vesical ligament is divided anteriorly (Figure 18.1). The bladder is then mobilised off the cervix and the **ureters displaced** upwards and laterally.

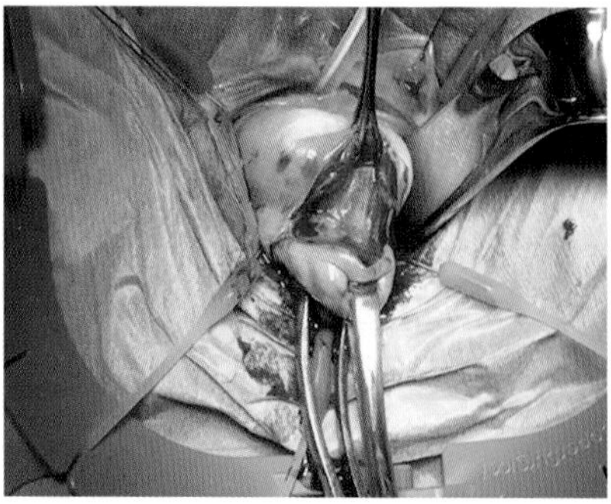

With upward traction on the cervix, the **peritoneum of the posterior cul-de-sac** is cut with Mayo scissors to access the **Pouch of Douglas (posterior colpotomy).** The colpotomy incision is stretched with both index fingers and a Sims speculum is gently placed to protect the rectum (Figure 18.2).

The **anterior uterovesical pouch** is then opened and the bladder and **ureters deflected from the field of surgery.** A curved **Gwilliams hysterectomy clamp** is applied to the **uterosacral** and **cardinal ligaments** at right angles to minimise ureteric injury. Avoid including too much tissue in the pedicle which may cause slippage. The pedicle is cut medial to the clamp and transfixed with a Vicryl 1 suture. This suture is usually kept long so that the uterosacral pedicle can be identified later. The process is repeated on the contralateral side. A further clamp may be used to secure the remainder of the cardinal ligaments. Some surgeons double ligate all pedicles to ensure total haemostasis and always

Figure 18.1 After an anterior vaginal incision, the bladder is held with Babcock forceps and mobilised off the cervix.

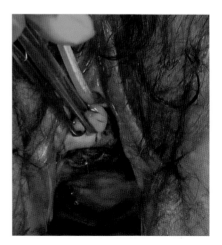

Figure 18.2 Posterior colpotomy incision to access the pouch of Douglas.

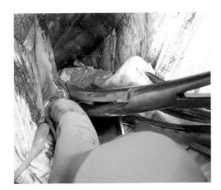

Figure 18.3 Curved Gwilliams clamp applied to uterine vessels which are then ligated.

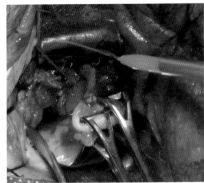

Figure 18.4 Left oophorectomy performed using an Endoloop ligature.

ensure that each successive clamp is placed medial to the previous pedicle.

The uterine vessels are clamped and then transfixed. For this vascular pedicle, the **curved Gwilliams clamp** is applied as close to the uterine body as possible (Figure 18.3). The suture is cut deliberately short to avoid inadvertent avulsion of uterine vessels.

If the ovaries are to be conserved, the round ligaments, ovarian ligaments and fallopian tubes are secured and ligated: this may need to be performed individually depending on the thickness of tissue. The ovaries are inspected and if they are to be removed, the infundibulopelvic (IP) ligaments are clamped, cut and transfixed. It is sometimes easier to complete the oophorectomy after removal of the uterus and cervix. In this video, **oophorectomy** was performed using a pre-tied **Ethicon Vicryl endoscopic loop** (Figure 18.4).

The **uterosacral ligaments** can be sutured to the posterior peritoneal edge and the **vaginal vault** to suspend the vault and **prevent enterocoele formation.** Ensure that all the pedicles are 'dry' before closing the vaginal vault with a continuous suture. As shown in this video, a **Redivac**

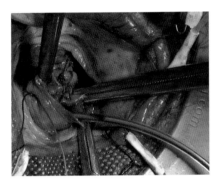

Figure 18.5 A Redivac drain being sited through the vaginal suture line for venous ooze.

drain can be inserted into the peritoneal cavity if there is venous ooze (Figure 18.5). The vaginal vault can also be packed if there is further ongoing venous ooze.

Summary of Procedure Steps

1 Grasp cervix with vulsellum forceps.
2 Infiltrate adrenaline with bupivacaine.
3 Incise circumferentially around the cervix.
4 Divide the cervico-vesical ligament.
5 Open the pouch of Douglas.
6 Clamp the uterosacral and cardinal ligaments bilaterally, cut and transfix.

7 Clamp the remainder of the cardinal ligaments bilaterally, cut and transfix (if required).

8 Open the uterovesical peritoneal pouch.

9 Clamp the uterine vessels bilaterally, cut and transfix.

10 Divide the IP ligaments and round ligaments (for oophorectomy).

OR

11 Divide the fallopian tube, ovarian ligaments and round ligaments (for ovarian preservation) and inspect the ovaries.

12 Remove the uterus and cervix.

13 Reinforce the uterosacral ligaments to the posterior peritoneal edge and lateral angles of the vaginal vault.

14 Check for haemostasis of the pedicles.

15 Close the vaginal vault.

Postoperative Care

1 If the Enhanced Recovery pathway is followed, bladder catheter and vaginal pack should be avoided: this encourages early mobilisation and possible discharge on the same day.

2 If a vaginal pack, indwelling catheter or drain have been inserted, remove these as early as feasibly to encourage mobilisation.

3 Thromboprophylaxis (as per local guideline).

Conclusion

Although this chapter discusses vaginal hysterectomy performed for uterine prolapse, the vaginal route for hysterectomy should also be considered in the non-prolapse uterus for indications such as menorrhagia or fibroid.

Further Reading

Aarts, J.W.M., Nieboer, T.E., Johnson, N. et al. (2015). Surgical approach to hysterectomy for benign gynaecological disease. *Cochrane Review* 12 https://www.cochrane.org/CD003677/MENSTR_surgical-approach-hysterectomy-benign-gynaecological-diseases.

American College of Obstetricians and Gynecologists (2017). Committee Opinion 701. Choosing the route of hysterectomy for benign disease. https://www.acog.org/Clinical-Guidance-and-Publications/Committee-Opinions/Committee-on-Gynecologic-Practice/Choosing-the-Route-of-Hysterectomy-for-Benign-Disease?IsMobileSet=false.

RCOG (2015). Recovering well. Information for you after a vaginal hysterectomy. www.rcog.org.uk/en/patients/patient-leaflets/vaginal-hysterectomy.

Yoong, W., Sivashanmugarajan, V., Relph, S. et al. (2014). Can enhanced recovery pathways improve outcomes of vaginal hysterectomy? Cohort control study. *J. Minim. Invasive Gynecol.* 21 (1): 83–89. https://doi.org/10.1016/j.jmig.2013.06.007. Epub 2013 Jul 10. PMID: 23850899.

19 Manchester Repair (Fothergill's Operation) for Cervical Prolapse

Dhanuson Dharmasena and Wai Yoong

Video Duration | 8 mins 58 secs

Overview

This uterus conserving procedure has sometimes been forgotten to the detriment of trainees. Manchester repair is at least as safe as vaginal hysterectomy with similar outcomes and therefore should be offered as an alternative in selected patients. The authors discuss the indications as well as potential complications of this minimally invasive historic technique. Counselling is important, especially the need for cerclage in future pregnancy and the risk of cervical stenosis leading to haematometra.

Introduction

This uterus preserving operation was first described by **Professor Donald** from Manchester in 1908 and later modified by his colleague, **Professor Fothergill,** also from the same city, thus conferring the procedure with the name of **Manchester Repair.** This operation was designed for women with second- and third-degree uterine descent with the advantage that it has a **shorter operating time,** is associated with **less morbidity** and has a **quicker recovery** period. The principle behind this procedure is to **amputate the elongated cervix** and **approximate the cardinal ligaments anterior to the cervix** in order to elevate and retract it backwards so that the uterus is both anteverted and supported. This procedure has **fallen out of fashion** but recent studies have shown it to be a superior operation compared to vaginal hysterectomy.

Indications

1 When the symptoms are due to vaginal prolapse associated with elongation of the (supravaginal) cervix.
2 Preservation of reproductive function.

How to Perform Operative Procedures in Obstetrics and Gynaecology, First Edition.
Edited by Wai Yoong, Abha Govind, and Wasim Lodhi.
© 2020 John Wiley & Sons Ltd. Published 2020 by John Wiley & Sons Ltd.
Companion website: www.wiley.com/go/yoong/obgyn

Steps

Composite steps of Manchester Repair:
1 Preliminary dilatation and curettage (D&C).
2 Amputation of the cervix.
3 Plication of Mackenrodt's ligaments in front of cervix.
4 Anterior colporrhaphy (if necessary).

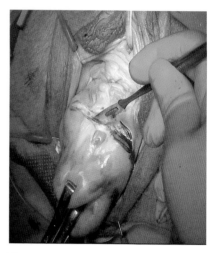

Figure 19.1 Full thickness circumferential cervical incision and mobilisation of the bladder.

Procedure

The uterus is initially **sounded** to establish cavity length and to confirm cervical elongation. The cervical canal is **dilated** to facilitate the passage of sutures through the canal during covering of the amputated cervix by vaginal flaps. Cervical dilatation also allows adequate uterine **drainage** and helps **prevent** cervical **stenosis** during healing of the external os. Endometrial **curettage** is often performed to sample the endometrium. Infiltrate with a solution of 20 ml of bupivacaine 0.5% w/v and adrenaline 1 : 200 000 circumferentially around the cervix.

The incision is as described for vaginal hysterectomy and repair. The vaginal skin is reflected circumferentially from the cervix (Figure 19.1) and the bladder mobilised from the cervix. Upwards traction of the posterior lip of the cervix using a vulsellum allows a pair of Allis forceps to be placed in the midpoint of the posterior cervicovaginal junction. The lateral and posterior vaginal wall is **dissected** off from the cervix by scissors and blunt dissection.

Mackenrodt's ligaments and the descending branch of the **uterine artery** are clamped on each side before being incised and tied (Figure 19.2). Any **enterocele** detected should be repaired. The

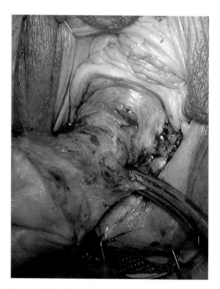

Figure 19.2 Mackenrodt's ligaments being clamped.

cervix is now **amputated** using a scalpel. The anterior lip of the amputated cervix is held with a vulsellum. A **Sturmdorff suture** is inserted to cover the posterior lip of the cervix with the vaginal flap.

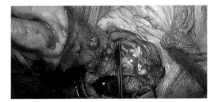

Figure 19.3 Elongated cervix being excised.

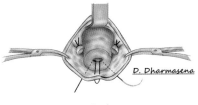

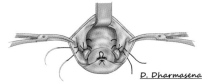

Figure 19.4 Insertion of Sturmdorff and Fothergill sutures. *Source*: Reproduced with permission of Dhanuson Dharmasena.

The Sturmdorff Suture

A Vicryl 1 suture is passed through the **posterior vaginal wall laterally** through the wall of the cervix into the **cervical canal** from which the needle is withdrawn to pick up the **mid-portion** of the posterior vaginal wall. The suture then **returns** to the cervical canal and out of the cervical **wall laterally** and through the vaginal wall (Figure 19.3). This Sturmdoff suture, when tied, **covers** the posterior portion of the amputated cervix.

Plication of Mackenrodt's Ligaments

The cut ends of Mackenrodt's ligaments are **sutured to the anterior surface** of the amputated cervix. Alternatively, the **Fothergill stitch** can be performed which allows the vaginal skin to cover the anterior portion of the amputated cervix and approximates the ligaments in front of it (Figure 19.4). The suture passes the vaginal wall laterally through **Mackenrodt's ligaments** and into the **cervical canal** from which it is withdrawn. The suture returns through the cervical canal and out of the anterior cervical wall to pass through the **contralateral** Mackenrodt's ligaments and finally exits finally through the vaginal wall.

Anterior Colporrhaphy

The **pubocervical fascia** is approximated as in an anterior colporrhaphy. The redundant portion of the vaginal mucosa is excised and the cut margins of the vagina are apposed together using a continuous suture. A posterior repair may be carried out if needed.

Complications

Complications following this surgery can be subdivided into three categories: intraoperative, postoperative and late complications. Intraoperative complications include **haemorrhage** and **injury to the bladder/rectum**. Postoperative complications include primary or secondary **haemorrhage, urinary tract infection** or localised **infection**. Late complications include **cervical stenosis** (leading to **haematometra**), **dyspareunia, cervical incompetency** and **cervical dystocia in labour**. Patients requiring preservation of fertility must be warned of the risk of cervical incompetence and preterm labour. An **elective cervical cerclage** must be offered to reduce this risk.

Further Reading

Donald, A. (1908). Operation in cases of complete prolapse. *J. Obstet. Gynaecol. Br. Emp.* 13: 195–196.

Fothergill, W.E. (1921). The end results of vaginal operations for genital prolapse. *J. Obstet. Gynaecol. Br. Emp.* 28: 251–255.

Tolstrup, C.K., Lose, G., and Klarskov, N. (2017). The Manchester procedure versus vaginal hysterectomy in the treatment of uterine prolapse: a review. *Int. Urogynecol. J.* 28 (1): 33–40.

20 Cone Biopsy

Jane Ding and Wai Yoong

Video Duration | 4 mins

Overview

Cone biopsy is a procedure that is not frequently performed or seen by obstetrics and gynaecology trainees. This chapter provides a brief overview of the procedure as well as the surgical steps and complications.

Introduction

Cone biopsy is not an operation frequently performed by junior gynaecologists. Trainees are likely to encounter these patients post-operatively with ongoing bleeding and, hence, need to understand the basic steps of the surgery involved. The purpose of this excisional technique is to remove a cone-shaped piece of cervical tissue which will include the entire **transformation zone,** for diagnosis as well as treatment. The indications for cone biopsy are: (i) 'see and treat' for severe **dyskaryosis** and (ii) cervical glandular intra-epithelial neoplasia (**CGIN),** and (iii) early invasive disease requiring **fertility preservation**.

Procedure

Cone biopsy cannot be performed as part of an outpatient colposcopy visit, due to the depth of the endocervical lesion or a suspicion of invasive disease. It is performed as a **day case** procedure under **general anaesthesia.** The patient is placed in lithotomy position and a Sims speculum is inserted. The cervix is visualised and **colposcopy** is performed. **Acetic acid** is applied to identify the limits of the lesion. Additional **Lugol's iodine** may be used.

A dental syringe containing a combination of **local anaesthetic** (e.g. lidocaine) and **vasoconstrictor agent** (e.g. adrenaline) such as Lignospan Special (20mg/ml and 12.5ug/ml) (Septodont Ltd) is used to infiltrate the cervix superficially at 3, 6, 9 and 12 o'clock areas (Figure 20.1). This helps to provide pain relief and reduce blood loss. A deep **haemostatic suture** is placed at each side of the cervix to ligate the descending cervical branch of the uterine artery, and to act as traction (Figure 20.2).

The cervix is held with a **vulsellum** and incised with a **scalpel** at an angle to the cervix to ensure an entire cone-shaped block of tissue is obtained (Figure 20.3).

How to Perform Operative Procedures in Obstetrics and Gynaecology, First Edition.
Edited by Wai Yoong, Abha Govind, and Wasim Lodhi.
© 2020 John Wiley & Sons Ltd. Published 2020 by John Wiley & Sons Ltd.
Companion website: www.wiley.com/go/yoong/obgyn

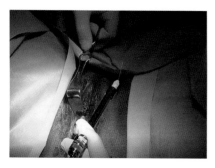

Figure 20.1   Infiltration using vasoconstrictor agents.

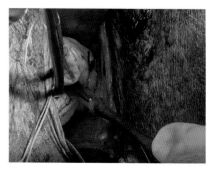

Figure 20.3   Excising a cone shaped segment of cervical tissue.

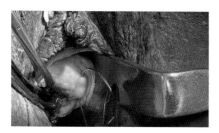

Figure 20.2   Ligating the descending cervical branch of the uterine vessels.

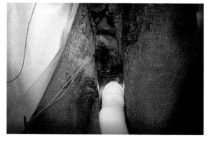

Figure 20.4   Cervical remnant prior to insertion of modified Sturmdorf suture.

It is best to **start** the incision **posteriorly** to allow the blood to run downwards and not obscure the visual field of the incision. The tissue is excised **circumferentially,** removed and sent for histology.

A **modified Sturmdorf suture** technique is used in this video for repair of the cervix (Figure 20.4). Please see Chapter 19 for more details. The **internal** cervical **os** must remain patent during the repair to allow normal flow of menstrual bleed. **Electrocautery** can be used to ensure haemostasis at raw edges. The ends of the haemostatic traction sutures are cut. Occasionally a vaginal pack and bladder catheter are left *in situ* to achieve haemostasis. The patient is asked to avoid vigorous exercise, swimming, use of a bath and heavy work for 48 hours. Most women are

able to go back to work within one or two weeks. They are asked to avoid using a tampon and sexual intercourse for four to six weeks after the cone biopsy.

Possible Risks

Cone biopsy carries a small risk of **heavy bleeding** and local sepsis. Antibiotics are needed if the patient complains of offensive vaginal discharge, persistent lower abdominal pain or high temperature. Very rarely **cervical stenosis** can lead to **haematometra.**

Pregnancy Risks

It is important to discuss the pregnancy risks in patients who undergo a cone biopsy, as there is a small increased risk of **mid-trimester miscarriage** and

preterm birth. Cervical length monitoring every two weeks is recommended from 16 weeks gestation.

Top Tips

1 Infiltrate the cervix with a local anaesthetic and vasoconstrictor.
2 Place lateral haemostatic traction sutures bilaterally.
3 Excise the cervix circumferentially.
4 Repair the cervix with modified Sturmdorf technique.
5 Check for haemostasis.

Further Reading

RCOG (2016). Reproductive Outcomes after Local Treatment for Preinvasive Cervical Disease. Scientific Impact Paper No. 21 July 2016. www.rcog.org.uk/globalassets/documents/guidelines/scientific-impact-papers/sip_21.pdf.

21 Rigid Cystoscopy

Wai Yoong

Video Duration | 2 mins 20 secs

Overview

Unless the trainee's rotation involves an attachment to a urogynaecologist, it is unlikely that he/she will get the opportunity to perform cystoscopy. This chapter explains how to do a rigid cystoscopy and a systematic method of inspecting the bladder.

Introduction

Cystoscopy refers to the endoscopic examination of the bladder and urethra and can either be done using a rigid or flexible cystoscope. For the gynaecologist, cystoscopy is routinely performed at the end of bladder operations, such as mid-urethral slings and colposuspension, or as part of surgery; for example, intravesical Botulinum injections or staging of gynaecological cancers.

Consent

Although a relatively safe and simple procedure, the gynaecologist needs to be aware of the risks of rigid cystoscopy and counsel the patient appropriately. The risks of cystoscopy in women include:

a mild transient burning or bleeding on passing urine;

b urinary tract infection;

c urinary retention requiring temporary insertion of a catheter;

d bleeding requiring removal of clots or further surgery;

e injury to the urethra and bladder.

Prophylactic Antibiotics

Little evidence is available regarding prophylactic antibiotics in diagnostic cystoscopy but women undergoing rigid cystoscopy should have a single intravenous dose of gentamycin at induction of anaesthesia.

Procedure and Equipment Preparation

We will focus mainly on **rigid cystoscopy** and how to do this procedure as gynaecologists are more likely to use rigid rather than flexible cystoscopy in their practice. The patient is positioned in the **lithotomy position** and prepared as for vaginal surgery. The cystoscope, which comprises the telescope, the outer sheath, obturator and bridge, is assembled. The **'0' of the bridge** is

How to Perform Operative Procedures in Obstetrics and Gynaecology, First Edition.
Edited by Wai Yoong, Abha Govind, and Wasim Lodhi.
© 2020 John Wiley & Sons Ltd. Published 2020 by John Wiley & Sons Ltd.
Companion website: www.wiley.com/go/yoong/obgyn

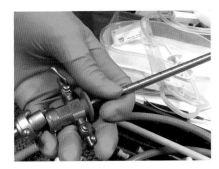

Figure 21.1   Aligning the '0' of the bridge to the '0' of the sheath.

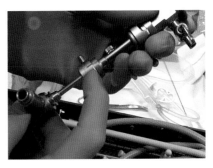

Figure 21.3   Inserting the cystoscope so that the '0's all align.

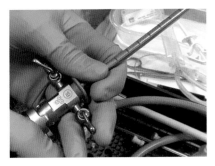

Figure 21.2   Locking the bridge to the sheath.

aligned to the **'0' of the sheath** (Figure 21.1) and the two parts are attached by **locking the lever** (Figure 21.2). The cystoscope is introduced such that the **'0' of the scope matches the '0' on the bridge** (Figure 21.3). For ergonomic reasons, it is preferable that the **irrigation channel** comes from the surgeon's **right-hand side,** whilst the **light lead, screen and stack** sits on the **left**: this helps avoid entangling the wires and saline giving sets. It is crucial that the distension medium is not pressurised as this can lead to overdistention or even rupture of the bladder.

How to Perform a Rigid Cystoscopy

Lubricant is applied along the cystoscope. The **visual obturator** and **a 30° lens** is used to enter the bladder. There is no single way of performing a cystoscopy but what is important is a systematic and thorough examination of the entire bladder.

One possible method is outlined below.

1 **Run the irrigation** through to avoid **excess bubbles** in the bladder.
2 Insert the cystoscope until the **obturator and lens is about 1 cm** within the urethra before starting irrigation: this prevents unnecessary spillage of distention fluid.
3 If there is significant debris, the bladder may need to be emptied by removing the telescope and visual obturator and using the outer sheath as a temporary catheter.
4 Note the colour, volume, debris or offensive smell of the urine. The bladder should be **sufficiently full (>250 ml)** to allow inspection of the walls. **Overfilling the bladder** should be avoided as this can distort the urothelium, making it harder to see subtle changes. This is especially crucial if biopsies are planned: overdistending the bladder makes the bladder wall thinner and more prone to injury.
5 Begin the examination by **visualising the dome** of the bladder. To do this, the surgeon's hands holding the cystoscope

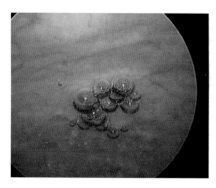

Figure 21.4 Visualising the 'bladder bubble' at the dome.

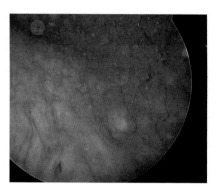

Figure 21.5 Visualising the ureteric orifices.

are gently lowered so that the tip of the telescope is pointing upwards. Ensure that the light lead is pointing downwards when using telescopes with angled lenses (30° or 70°). The **'bladder bubble'** should be visible at the dome and this helps with orientation (Figure 21.4).

6 The light lead can be rotated to face upwards so that **trigone and inter-ureteric bar** can be inspected. The cystoscope can then be turned to inspect the **left and right ureteric orifices** (Figure 21.5) by following the inter-ureteric bar.

TIP: The camera cable should hang downwards perpendicular to the floor and the cystoscope and light lead (not the camera) rotated to examine the bladder.

The bladder should be systematically assessed in **four quadrants,** taking into account diverticulum, bladder tumours/growths, petechiae (especially on refill) and trabeculation.

The **uretheric orifices** are usually located at **5 and 7 o'clock,** and **ureteric**

peristalsis and occasionally a spurt of urine can be seen being propelled from the orifices.

TIP: Remember that the patient may have an undiagnosed duplex kidney(s). Be alert to the possibility of finding more than two ureteric orifices at cystoscopy.

To examine the **anterior wall of the bladder,** the non-dominant (free) hand can be used to apply some pressure to the abdominal wall as the cystoscope is rotated to point upwards. In some cases, it may be necessary to empty the bladder to visualise the anterior wall near the dome. Lastly, as the telescope is withdrawn from the bladder, turn the irrigation back on and examine the urethra for any abnormalities such as **urethral diverticulum.**

Before removing the cystoscope, empty the bladder as this will make the patient more comfortable postoperatively.

Further Reading

Lyttle, M. and Fowler, G. (2017). Cystoscopy for the gynaecologist: how to do a cystoscopy. *Obstet. Gynaecol.* 19: 236–240.

22 Manual Vacuum Aspiration and Surgical Management of Miscarriage

Abha Govind and Beena Subba

Video Duration | 4 mins 21 secs

Overview

This chapter discusses manual vacuum aspiration (MVA) and suction curettage for retained products of conception, which are two basic mandatory competencies.

Introduction

Treatment options for miscarriage include **expectant, surgical** and **medical** management. Over the last few decades, MVA has emerged as an effective and safe alternative for surgical management of miscarriage.

Surgical management of miscarriage involves **suction evacuation** under general anaesthesia using **electric vacuum aspiration** (EVA). MVA can be carried out in the outpatient setting under local anaesthesia and was first described by **Harvey Karman,** who designed the vacuum syringe and defined the principles of MVA for surgical uterine evacuation.

MVA is also recommended as an effective and acceptable surgical method of termination of pregnancy in the Royal College of Obstetricians and Gynaecologists (RCOG) evidence-based guideline 'The care of women requesting induced abortion'.

Indication

MVA has been used for first-trimester termination of pregnancy, incomplete miscarriage, missed miscarriage, endometrial biopsy and following failed medical termination of pregnancy.

How to Perform Operative Procedures in Obstetrics and Gynaecology, First Edition.
Edited by Wai Yoong, Abha Govind, and Wasim Lodhi.
© 2020 John Wiley & Sons Ltd. Published 2020 by John Wiley & Sons Ltd.
Companion website: www.wiley.com/go/yoong/obgyn

MVA Syringe

MVA involves the use of a hand-held syringe as a source of suction instead of an electric suction machine. The syringe is made of latex-free plastic and can be single- or double-valved. The **double-valved** syringe is the updated version that is used more frequently. This has a volume of 60 ml and can create a vacuum of 610–660 mmHg.

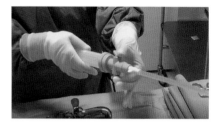

Figure 22.1 The MVA syringe is 'charged' by pressing the two valves.

Cannulae are 24 cm long and are colour-coded according to their diameter, which range from 4 mm to 12 mm. The size of the cannula is chosen according to **gestation** and the estimated size of the uterus. It has **graduations** with six markers starting at 6 cm from the tip and spaced 1 cm apart. The tube is flexible and the tips are rounded to help minimise the risk of uterine perforation.

Procedure

MVA can be performed in the early pregnancy assessment unit **(EPAU)**. Written **consent** should be obtained, and the cervix can be prepared with synthetic prostaglandin E_1 (misoprostol 400 μg), two to three hours prior to the procedure, especially in women with a tightly closed cervix.

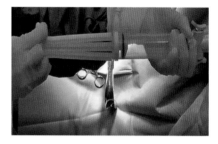

Figure 22.2 The plunger is pulled back to create a vacuum.

Pain relief can be provided with 500 mg naproxen or 400–800 mg ibuprofen given orally one hour before the procedure. In women with contraindications to non-steroidal anti-inflammatory drugs, paracetamol and/or codeine can be used.

Baseline **observations** of pulse, temperature and blood pressure are taken on admission. The patient is asked to empty her bladder just before the procedure. **Vaginal examination** is performed after cleaning and draping, with the woman in the **lithotomy** position. The size and position of the uterus and cervix are then assessed.

The MVA syringe is **charged** by pressing **distal valves** of the syringe until they click into the locking position (Figure 22.1). The **plunger** is then pulled backwards to generate a vacuum until it eventually locks (Figure 22.2). Lidocaine hydrochloride 2% anaesthetic gel can be applied topically to the cervix, followed by a paracervical injection of local anaesthetic (30 mg/ml prilocaine and 0.03 IU/ml felypressin) into the four quadrants using a dental needle (0.40 × 35 mm, 27 G).

The anterior lip of the cervix is held with an Allis forceps and an appropriately sized cannula is introduced into the uterus. If required, the cervical os is gently dilated with the rounded tip of the cannula or, alternatively, **Hegar dilators** can be used. The charged syringe is then attached to the cannula. The proximal valves on the syringe are released and the operator moves the syringe in a rotating motion in the uterus, aspirating intrauterine contents into the syringe. After the syringe is about **80% full** with products of conception, it is detached from the cannula and the contents emptied into a bowl. The syringe is charged again and reattached to the cannula and the **process repeated** until the uterine cavity is empty. The woman can then recover in an easy chair and should be allowed to go home within one or two hours after completion of the procedure.

The outpatient department should be equipped with **emergency resuscitation** equipment including intravenous cannulae, intravenous fluids, adrenaline (epinephrine), oxygen, atropine, oxytocin, misoprostol and a defibrillator, to handle common medical emergencies.

Careful **case selection** of low-risk women (multiparous, well-motivated, CRL <25mm, incomplete miscarriage with retained products of conception <5cm and haemodynamically stable) can reduce the chance of unexpected emergencies.

Women with >10 weeks gestation, those who are anxious, those with cervical stenosis, fibroids uterus or bleeding disorders are not suitable for outpatient MVA and should have a suction evacuation of products of conception under GA.

Suction curettage is a surgical procedure in which the cervix is dilated and a suction cannula used to remove the products of conception from the uterine cavity.

The legs are positioned in lithotomy position and a Sims speculum inserted into the vagina. The cervix is held with a velsellum and **dilated** with Hegar dilators to allow insertion of an instrument. A laminaria (Dilapan®) or misoprostol 400 µg two hours prior to the procedure often helps to soften and ripen the cervix.

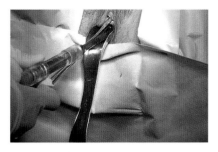

Figure 22.3 Suction curette being introduced through the cervix following dilatation.

As a general rule, a Hegar size 7 dilator is used to dilate the cervix in a seven-week pregnancy, i.e. the dilator size corresponding approximately to pregnancy gestation in weeks. A suction **cannula** is then introduced through the cervix and products of conception removed by rotating the mouth of the cannula through 360° starting at the fundus (Figure 22.3). Sharp and blunt curettage using a standard curette is performed to ensure that the cavity is completely empty. The tissue removed then goes for a **histological** examination. Common **side effects** include cramping, spotting or light bleeding. Damage to the cervix and perforation of the uterus or bladder and blood vessels are rare. Advise the patient to report heavy or prolonged bleeding or blood clots, fever, pain, abdominal tenderness or foul-smelling discharge from the vagina. In very rare cases, adhesions may form inside the uterus causing Asherman's syndrome. This may cause infertility and changes in menstrual flow.

Recovery After Surgical Management of Miscarriage

After suction curettage, one can return to regular activities within one or two days. One can expect a change in the timing of the next menstrual period. It may come either early or late. If any tissue was sent for a biopsy, the result is usually available within several days.

Further Reading

Karman, H. and Potts, M. (1972). Very early abortion using syringe as vacuum source. *Lancet* 1: 1051–1052.

RCOG (2011). The care of women requesting induced abortion: Evidence-based Green-top Guideline No. 7.

Sharma, M. (2015). Manual vacuum aspiration: an outpatient alternative for surgical management of miscarriage. *Obstet. Gynaecol.* 17: 157–161.

23 Female Sterilisation: The Laparoscopic and Hysteroscopic Approaches

Abha Govind

Video Duration 5 mins 11 secs

Overview

Female sterilisation is performed to **permanently** prevent pregnancy. The fallopian tubes are occluded to prevent the egg and sperm meeting, and this is more than 99% effective in preventing pregnancy. The procedure is usually undertaken laparoscopically but can also be done hysteroscopically or as an open procedure. The video accompanying this chapter shows laparoscopic tubal occlusion using **Filshie clips** as well as the hysteroscopic approach using an **Essure** device (Bayer AG). Hysteroscopic sterilisation was still being practised when this video chapter was filmed, but Essure has been withdrawn by its company, Bayer AG in 2018. The editors have decided to include it for historic interest.

Laparoscopic Clip Sterilisation

The laparoscopic procedure is usually done under general anaesthesia (GA) but can be done under regional block. Blocking or removal of the fallopian tubes is effective immediately. The patient needs to **continue using contraception** up until the operation, and until her next period. The **risks** of laparoscopic sterilisation are same as those of diagnostic laparoscopy, i.e. a small risk of bleeding, infection or damage to the bowel or bladder. There is a 1 : 200 risk of **failure** either due to the clip being applied on the wrong structure (round or ovarian ligaments) or due to recanalisation of the blocked tubes. If the operation fails, this may increase the risk of a fertilised egg implanting in the fallopian tube leading to an **ectopic pregnancy.** Sterilisation is very difficult to reverse, and reversal operations are rarely funded by the NHS. The preoperative **consent,** therefore, has to be taken

How to Perform Operative Procedures in Obstetrics and Gynaecology, First Edition.
Edited by Wai Yoong, Abha Govind, and Wasim Lodhi.
© 2020 John Wiley & Sons Ltd. Published 2020 by John Wiley & Sons Ltd.
Companion website: www.wiley.com/go/yoong/obgyn

with care. The woman needs to be counselled that sterilisation does not protect against sexually transmitted infections (STIs) and she will need to use condoms as well.

Consent

Almost any woman can be sterilised, but it should only be considered by those who do not want any more children or do not want children at all. As sterilisation is permanent, all options of **long acting reversible methods of contraception (LARC)** and **vasectomy** must be discussed. The woman is more likely to be accepted for sterilisation if she is **over 30** and has had children. Woman sterilised before the age of 30 may **regret** having the procedure. Some general practitioners and family planning clinics will offer counselling before referring the woman to secondary care for sterilisation. **Counselling** gives a chance to talk about the operation in detail and discuss any doubts, worries or questions.

Where possible, the woman and her partner should both agree to the procedure, but it is not a legal requirement to get the partner's permission. The consent should include a **mini-laparotomy** if the laparoscopic procedure could not be completed. This sometimes occurs in women who have had previous abdominal or pelvic surgery or pelvic inflammatory disease, causing adhesions, or in the morbidly obese.

Steps of Laparoscopic Clip Female Sterilisation

A **pregnancy test** should be to undertaken prior to sterilisation, which can be performed at any stage of the menstrual cycle. The procedure is undertaken as a **day case** under GA. As part of documentation, the surgeon should include **images** in the patient's notes confirming the site and correct application on the tube. In cases of complete or partial salpingectomy, the excised fallopian tube should be sent for **histology** as evidence that the procedure has been successfully undertaken.

1 Place the patient in the dorsal lithotomy position.
2 Empty the bladder with a urinary catheter.
3 Insert a Spackman's uterine manipulator.
4 Obtain laparoscopic access to the peritoneal cavity (Veress needle, direct trocar entry, open laparoscopic technique).
5 Place the laparoscope into the trocar and confirm correct placement in the abdominal cavity by systematically surveying the anatomy. Then, view directly under the trocar site to confirm there is no injury to the omentum or small bowel.
6 View the uterus, ovaries, and fallopian tubes by pushing the uterine manipulator upwards and anteriorly ('anteverting the uterus'). Inspect the pouch of Douglas, the uterosacral ligaments and the ovarian fossa. Document the visual appearance of the appendix, liver and the under surface of the diaphragm and gallbladder.
7 It is important that the fallopian tube is clearly identified. Follow the fallopian tubes from the uterine cornu to the fimbrial ends on each side. Identify the round ligament.
8 Identify a preferred location for the second trocar. Left iliac fossa or suprapubic sites are generally preferred. Identify anatomical landmarks to avoid the bladder and inferior epigastric arteries.

Tubal Ligation Technique

Tubal ligation technique varies with the chosen method, as described below.

Filshie Clip

1 This involves applying a titanium clip with silicone rubber lining around the fallopian tube. The Filshie clip works by exerting continued pressure, causing avascular necrosis of the 3 to 5 mm of the tube where it was applied. Fibrosis then occurs, and the clip is peritonealised.

2 The applicator is placed though a 7 or 8 mm trocar in the second port.

3 The Filshie clip is loaded onto its applicator with its jaws initially open (Figure 23.1). To fit it through the port, the jaws are closed partially by compressing the applicator handle halfway. Take care not to close the clip completely. Once the end of the applicator is in the abdomen, pressure on the handle is released in order to open the jaws of the clip.

4 Anteversion using the uterine manipulator helps to improve visualisation and access by straightening the fallopian tube.

5 The clip is placed perpendicular to the isthmic portion of the tube, about 2 cm from the cornu, so that the jaws completely encompass the tube (Figure 23.2). Avoid pulling on the fallopian tube during the application as this can cause avulsion.

6 The clip should then be partially closed by pressing the handle halfway to ensure that it is correctly placed. The applicator may be gently twisted to ensure that the tube is completely occluded.

7 Once the clip is placed correctly, slowly compress the handle completely – count to 5 until the fallopian tube blanches and the jaws of the clip are seen overlapping in the mesosalpinx. Release the clip by relaxing on the handle and carefully withdraw from the fallopian tube.

Finishing the Procedure

Perform the procedure on the contralateral tube. Remove the lateral and suprapubic ports under direct supervision. For trocar sites of 10 mm or more, reapproximate the rectus sheath using a J shaped needle. The skin incisions can be closed with 2/0 vicryl or an absorbable monofilament suture (4–0). Remove the uterine manipulator and inspect the cervix for any bleeding. An injection of 2 ml of 0.5% bupivacaine at the port sites can decrease postoperative pain.

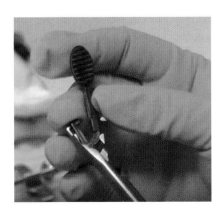

Figure 23.1 Filshie clip loaded into the applicator with its jaws open.

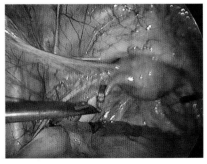

Figure 23.2 Bilateral placement of Filshie clips approximately 2 cm from cornu.

Pomeroy Procedure (Partial Salpingectomy)

Tubal ligation can be undertaken through a mini-laparotomy using the **Pomeroy's technique** (partial salpingectomy) as an interval procedure. A Spencer-Wells forceps is used to pull a loop of the fallopian tube away from the blood vessels in the mesosalpinx. The loop is tied with 2/0 vicryl suture. The looped portion of the fallopian tube is excised with the Mcindoe's scissors. A minimum of 1 cm segment of the tube should be removed to decrease the failure rate. The excised tubal segments are sent for histology.

Salpingectomy

If occlusion of the fallopian tube has not worked, the tube can be excised (salpingectomy). A laparoscopic salpingectomy can be performed using monopolar scissors, a Harmonic scalpel or endoscopic loop to achieve sterilisation. This technique is explained in more detail in Chapter 16.

Essure Hysteroscopic Sterilisation

The Essure device was licenced by the Food and Drug Administration of the United States Department of Health and Human Services in 2002. It was eventually withdrawn from use by the parent company, Bayer AG in 2018. **Essure** uses soft, **flexible inserts** placed in the fallopian tubes using a hysteroscopic approach. In the three months following insertion, the device induces luminal fibrosis, leading to tubal occlusion. During this time the patient must continue using another form of contraception to prevent a pregnancy.

Essure placement requires a Bettocchi hysteroscope system and can be performed in a hysteroscopy suite. Patient can take analgesia to reduce anxiety. The Essure system has two components: a micro-insert and a delivery catheter. The **micro-insert** comprises a spring-like device which is 40 mm in length and 0.8 mm in diameter (Figure 23.3). The micro-insert has an inner coil made of stainless steel, a nickel titanium (nitinol) elastic outer coil and polyethylene fibres. When released from the **delivery system,** the outer coil expands to 2.0 mm to anchor the micro-insert into the fallopian tube. The device is deployed using a continuous flow hysteroscope with a '5' French operating channel. **Optimal placement** is described as insertion with minimal resistance with three to eight coils left trailing in the uterine cavity (Figure 23.4). The majority of women return to normal activity within 24 hours and the procedure is 99.3% effective at preventing a pregnancy.

Essure was designed as an alternative to laparoscopic tubal ligation. A 2009 review concluded that Essure appeared safe and effective based on short-term studies; furthermore, it was less invasive and more cost effective than laparoscopic bilateral tubal ligation. Initial trials found that 4% women had tubal perforation, expulsion or misplacement of the device

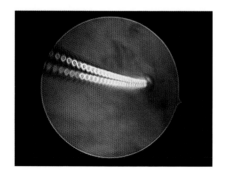

Figure 23.3 Essure device approaching the uterine ostia prior to deployment.

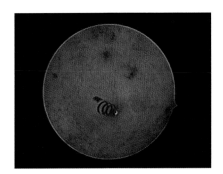

Figure 23.4 Correct placement of deployed device with 3–8 coils in the uterine cavity.

at the time of the procedure. However, later studies showed that the rates of repeat surgery in the first year were 10 times greater with Essure than with traditional tubal ligation. Bayer AG announced the cessation of sales in the United States by the end of 2018.

Further Reading

Murthy, P., Edwards, J., and Pathak, M. (2017). Update on hysteroscopic sterilisation. *Obstet. Gynaecol.* 19: 227–235. 10.1111/tog.12390.

RCOG (2016). Female sterilisation consent advise No. 3. www.rcog.org.uk/en/guidelines-research-services/guidelines/consent-advice-3.

RCOG (n.d.). E learning: https://elearning.rcog.org.uk//minimal-access-surgery/laparoscopic-procedures/laparoscopic-sterilisation.

Index

Page locators in **bold** indicate tables. Page locators in *italics* indicate figures.

How to Perform Operative Procedures in Obstetrics and Gynaecology, First Edition.
Edited by Wai Yoong, Abha Govind, and Wasim Lodhi.
© 2020 John Wiley & Sons Ltd. Published 2020 by John Wiley & Sons Ltd.
Companion website: www.wiley.com/go/yoong/obgyn